I0036620

# Orofacial and Systemic Features of Thalassemia Major: Management, and Prevention with Reference to Populations in the Arabian Gulf

Authored by

## Faiez N. Hattab

*Visiting Professor of Pediatric Dentistry*
*Munich*
*Germany*

**Orofacial and Systemic Features of Thalassemia Major: Management, and Prevention with Reference to Populations in the Arabian Gulf**

Author: Faiez N. Hattab

ISBN (Online): 978-1-68108-814-3

ISBN (Print): 978-1-68108-815-0

ISBN (Paperback): 978-1-68108-816-7

© 2021, Bentham Books imprint.

Published by Bentham Science Publishers – Sharjah, UAE. All Rights Reserved.

# BENTHAM SCIENCE PUBLISHERS LTD.
## End User License Agreement (for non-institutional, personal use)

This is an agreement between you and Bentham Science Publishers Ltd. Please read this License Agreement carefully before using the ebook/echapter/ejournal (**"Work"**). Your use of the Work constitutes your agreement to the terms and conditions set forth in this License Agreement. If you do not agree to these terms and conditions then you should not use the Work.

Bentham Science Publishers agrees to grant you a non-exclusive, non-transferable limited license to use the Work subject to and in accordance with the following terms and conditions. This License Agreement is for non-library, personal use only. For a library / institutional / multi user license in respect of the Work, please contact: permission@benthamscience.net.

## Usage Rules:

1. All rights reserved: The Work is the subject of copyright and Bentham Science Publishers either owns the Work (and the copyright in it) or is licensed to distribute the Work. You shall not copy, reproduce, modify, remove, delete, augment, add to, publish, transmit, sell, resell, create derivative works from, or in any way exploit the Work or make the Work available for others to do any of the same, in any form or by any means, in whole or in part, in each case without the prior written permission of Bentham Science Publishers, unless stated otherwise in this License Agreement.
2. You may download a copy of the Work on one occasion to one personal computer (including tablet, laptop, desktop, or other such devices). You may make one back-up copy of the Work to avoid losing it.
3. The unauthorised use or distribution of copyrighted or other proprietary content is illegal and could subject you to liability for substantial money damages. You will be liable for any damage resulting from your misuse of the Work or any violation of this License Agreement, including any infringement by you of copyrights or proprietary rights.

## Disclaimer:

Bentham Science Publishers does not guarantee that the information in the Work is error-free, or warrant that it will meet your requirements or that access to the Work will be uninterrupted or error-free. The Work is provided "as is" without warranty of any kind, either express or implied or statutory, including, without limitation, implied warranties of merchantability and fitness for a particular purpose. The entire risk as to the results and performance of the Work is assumed by you. No responsibility is assumed by Bentham Science Publishers, its staff, editors and/or authors for any injury and/or damage to persons or property as a matter of products liability, negligence or otherwise, or from any use or operation of any methods, products instruction, advertisements or ideas contained in the Work.

## Limitation of Liability:

In no event will Bentham Science Publishers, its staff, editors and/or authors, be liable for any damages, including, without limitation, special, incidental and/or consequential damages and/or damages for lost data and/or profits arising out of (whether directly or indirectly) the use or inability to use the Work. The entire liability of Bentham Science Publishers shall be limited to the amount actually paid by you for the Work.

## General:

1. Any dispute or claim arising out of or in connection with this License Agreement or the Work (including non-contractual disputes or claims) will be governed by and construed in accordance with the laws of Singapore. Each party agrees that the courts of the state of Singapore shall have exclusive jurisdiction to settle any dispute or claim arising out of or in connection with this License Agreement or the Work (including non-contractual disputes or claims).
2. Your rights under this License Agreement will automatically terminate without notice and without the

need for a court order if at any point you breach any terms of this License Agreement. In no event will any delay or failure by Bentham Science Publishers in enforcing your compliance with this License Agreement constitute a waiver of any of its rights.

3. You acknowledge that you have read this License Agreement, and agree to be bound by its terms and conditions. To the extent that any other terms and conditions presented on any website of Bentham Science Publishers conflict with, or are inconsistent with, the terms and conditions set out in this License Agreement, you acknowledge that the terms and conditions set out in this License Agreement shall prevail.

**Bentham Science Publishers Ltd.**
Executive Suite Y - 2
PO Box 7917, Saif Zone
Sharjah, U.A.E.
Email: subscriptions@benthamscience.net

**BENTHAM SCIENCE**

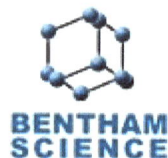

# CONTENTS

# FOREWORD

I am very pleased to write a foreword to this special monograph **"Orofacial and Systemic Features of Thalassemia Major: Management, and Prevention with Reference to Populations in the Arabian Gulf "**, by Dr. Faiez N. Hattab, a friend and colleague for more than 30 years. Thalassemia is a growing global public health problem with severe social impact in which few data are available in the populations of the Arabian Gulf region. This monograph provides an outstanding source of current information on thalassemia focusing on practical clinical approaches to the features, physiopathology, complications and management of the disease. It will provide valuable assistance to dental and clinical practitioners, especially those working in multiracial communities.

**Nasser Fouda**
Senior Consultant of Periodontics
UAE

# PREFACE

Thalassemia is one of the most common genetic diseases in the world. In high incidence areas, particularly Mediterranean and Middle Eastern countries, it presents a major public health and social challenge. This monograph updates dental and orofacial characteristics of thalassemia major. The clinical, radiographical, and odontometric features are also presented. Pathogenesis, systemic complications, morbidity and mortality, management, and prevention methods are discussed. Furthermore, guidelines for optimal dental care are also presented. The monograph contains the following key topics: introduction, epidemiology, consanguinity, pathophysiology, clinical and hematologic diagnosis, genetic testing, dental and orofacial features, literature review, mode of treatment, morbidity and mortality, diet and nutrition, cost of treatment, prevention, dental care, and genetic disorders in Arabian Gulf populations and among Arabs. Dental and orofacial characteristics include (i) maxillofacial deformities; (ii) dental caries and periodontal status; (iii) tooth size and dental arches dimensions; (iv) occlusion; (v) dental development;(vi) physical growth. The monograph contains 95 pages, 16 colored photographs, 15 radiographs, 4 drawings, 4 tables, and 2 plates. I hope this work will be helpful to dental and medical students, practitioners, and health educators, to update their knowledge about the nature of the disease.

**CONSENT FOR PUBLICATION**

Not applicable.

**CONFLICT OF INTEREST**

The author declares no conflict of interest, financial or otherwise.

**ACKNOWLEDGEMENTS**

I would like to thank Mr. Najwan F. Hattab for excellent proofreading the monograph.

**Faiez Najeeb Hattab**
Visiting Professor of Pediatric Dentistry
Munich
Germany

## ABSTRACT

Thalassemia is a group of hereditary hemoglobinopathies. It is one of the most common genetic disorders worldwide, presenting major public health and social challenges in high incidence areas. Thalassemia is inherited in an autosomal recessive manner. It is manifested as chronic hemolytic anemia, which is caused by partial or complete lack of the synthesis of alpha- or beta-globulin chains that form hemoglobin. Thalassemia major (TM) is associated with the most serious clinical changes and life-threatening risk and is characterized by the triad of chronic anemia, ineffective erythropoiesis, and iron overload. Anemia can be treated with regular blood transfusions, but this life-saving therapy results in a "second disease" due to iron accumulation in the body tissues. Iron overload is the main cause of morbidity and mortality. The oral and maxillofacial features of TM are protruding frontal and malar bones, thinning of the mandibular inferior cortex, small maxillary sinuses, maxillary hypertrophy, and flaring of the maxillary anterior teeth. Dental complications of TM include dental caries, periodontal disease, reduction in tooth size, teeth spacing, short and narrow dental arches, delayed tooth development, malocclusion. This monograph discusses the epidemiology, pathophysiology, clinical manifestations, radiological characteristics, dental care, management and complications. Guidelines for dental care are presented and stratiges of thalassemia prevention are reviewed.

**Keywords**: Clinical features, Complications, Consanguinity, Epidemiology, Management, Pathophysiology, Prevention, Thalassemia.

## INTRODUCTION

The term thalassemia is derived from the Greek "Thalassa" (sea) and "haima" (blood), as the disorder was first identified in the Mediterranean area. Thalassemia refers to a group of inherited hemolytic anemia disorders that involve defects in the synthesis of hemoglobin (Hb). Normal red blood cells (RBCs) each contain approximately 300 million molecules of Hb. In adults, there are three main types of Hb molecule: HbA, which on average represents around 96% of the Hb; HbA2, which is approximately 3%, and HbF, which is approximately 1%. Each HbA molecule consists of four globin chains, two α alpha and two β beta, associated with the central heme group of porphyrin ring and ferrous iron (Fig. **1a**) that can reversibly bind one oxygen molecule. The α chain has 141 amino acids and the β chain has 146 amino acids, arranged in a definite order. Mutation in globin genes

**Faiez N. Hattab**
**All rights reserved-© 2021 Bentham Science Publishers**

(11p15.5) causes a defect in the formation of α- or β-polypeptide. Alpha thalassemia occurs when one or more of the α-globin genes are affected, while β-thalassemia occurs when both β-globin genes are defective [1-3]. A decrease in the synthesis of globin leads to reduced Hb production, hypochromic microcytic anemia, and dysplastic RBCs (erythrocytes) of deficit Hb content (Fig. **1b**). About 1540 variants of the globin gene sequence have been identified. More than 200 mutations have been identified in β-thalassemia. About 1540 variants of the globin gene sequence have been identified. More than 200 mutations have been identified in β-thalassemia [4]. These mutations can interact to produce a wide range of clinical and hematological phenotypes of variable severity from silent to very severe. The manifestations of thalassemia are regulated by a variety of genetic, racial, and environmental factors [2-5].

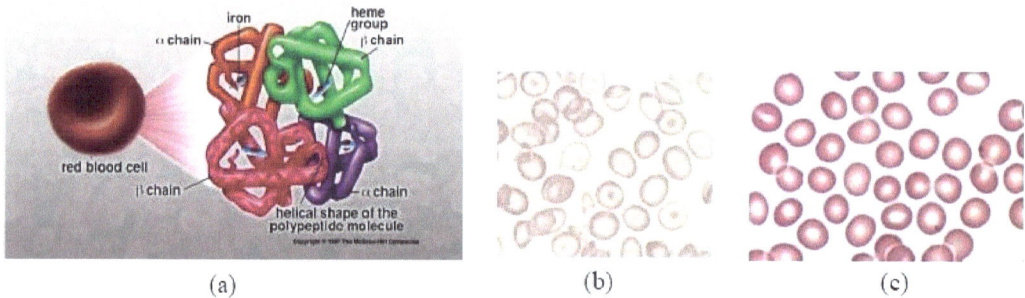

Fig. (1). (a) Normal hemoglobin structure made of heme, α globins, and β globins. (b) RBCs in thalassemia major are microcytic, hypochromic (pale), fragmented, and poikilocyte (abnormal shaped). (c) Normal RBCs [Source: *Google Images*].

## CLASSIFICATION OF THALASSEMIA

According to potential genetic defects and clinical severity, thalassemia is divided into two main diseases: α-thalassemia and β-thalassemia. It is also divided into transfusion-dependent and non-transfusion-dependent thalassemias. This classification is based on whether the patient requires regular blood transfusions to survive or not. Thalassemia covers α-thalassemia, β-thalassemia, and combinations of the two. Due to the differences in chain production and severity of symptoms, both α- and β-thalassemia are divided into minor or major, in addition to a variety of intermediates.

## Alpha Thalassemia

Alpha-globins production is regulated by four α-genes. Alpha-thalassemia is usually caused by a reduction (α+) or completely abolished (α°) globin chains production by the affected allele. The carrier state can either be α+ trait (α-thalassemia 2) or be α°-trait (α-thalassemia 1). It is one of the most common Hb genetic abnormalities, caused by one or more deletions or mutations in the four α-globin gene copies. α-thalassemia is characterized by a decrease in the amount of normal Hb, so there is insufficient oxygen in the body tissues. Affected individuals are suffering from RBCs deficiency, weakness, fatigue, yellowing of the skin, and complications of anemia. This form of the disease is widespread in tropical and subtropical regions. The more genes are affected, the less α-globin is produced. There are at least 4 different types of α-thalassemia, classified according to the number of genes affected and to the pathologic severity, including:

●Silent carrier (1 gene affected). People who have mutations in only one α-globin gene are silent carriers. They usually have normal Hb levels and RBC index with no signs or symptoms. DNA analysis is the only method to identify a silent carrier.

● Alpha thalassemia trait (2 genes affected, also called α-thalassemia minor). In this form, only one α-globin gene is dysfunctional, the RBCs are mildly microcytic, hypochromic, decrease in mean corpuscular volume. It is an asymptomatic carrier state but can be associated with mild chronic anemia that does not respond to iron supplements. Carriers usually do not require any treatment.

●Hemoglobin H disease (3 genes affected). This form of α-thalassemia is most common in people of Southeast Asian and Mediterranean descent. In this disease, the production of α-globin chains is significantly reduced, resulting in excessive β chains (HbH disease, also known as α-thalassemia intermedia). It can cause mild to moderate anemia, which is characterized by microcytic hypochromic hemolytic anemia, mild jaundice, splenomegaly, and bone deformities. For HbH disease, only occasional blood transfusions are usually required. Iron overload during the course of blood transfusions must be treated with iron chelators.

●Alpha thalassemia major (also called hydrops fetalis). This is the most severe form of α-thalassemia caused by the deletion of all four α-globin genes. Thus, normal Hb will not be produced. More than 20 different genetic mutations that result in the functional deletion of both pairs of α-globin genes have been identified. This situation is incompatible with life. Fetuses affected by α-thalassemia major have anemia in the first trimester. Clinical signs and symptoms include severe anemia, enlarged liver and spleen, extramedullary erythropoiesis, hydrocephalus, heart and urogenital defects, and retention of excess fluids (hydropic). Most babies with this condition are stillborn or die shortly after birth. Bone marrow transplant has helped to cure a small number of individuals with severe α-thalassemia.

## Beta Thalassemia

Different types of β-thalassemia gene mutations will produce different clinical and hematological phenotypes, the severity of which ranges from clinically asymptomatic to severe anemia. β-thalassemia is divided into three main forms according to the severity: thalassemia minor (trait), thalassemia intermedia, and thalassemia major (TM), with several subtypes of different clinical characteristics [2-5]. Due to its genetic heterogeneity, β-thalassemia is classified as homozygous, heterozygous, or compound heterozygous . Heterozygous β-thalassemia minor ($\beta^{++}$) is caused by mutations in one Hb β-gene with a minimal deficit in β-globin synthesis, which is not enough to cause problems in the normal functioning of the Hb. Carriers of this condition are usually clinically asymptomatic and have no health problems except for possible mild anemia. Mutations in the two β-genes result in a severe reduction of β-globin chains (β-thalassemia intermedia, $\beta^+$) or lack in β-globin production (β-thalassemia major, $\beta^0$). The homozygous β-thalassemia major is associated with the most severe signs and symptoms of other types of thalassemia.

### Beta Thalassemia Minor

Minor β-thalassemia is a defect in the synthesis of the β-chain of hemoglobin due to a mutation in the β-globin gene. The disorder is more prevalent among populations of African, Mediterranean and Southeast Asian countries. Most patients with minor β-thalassemia have mild anemia, which may be confused with iron deficiency anemia. Affected individuals do not have any serious medical problems; most of them may not even be aware that they have the disease. In thalassemia minor, RBCs are microcytic, hypochromic, and have decreased Hb levels. The signs and symptoms of the disease include mild anemia, tiredness, and weakness, or they may be absent. In some cases, enlargement of the spleen and hemolysis may occur. The disease usually does not require treatment. Folic acid supplementation is recommended. Iron supplementation is neither required nor recommended.

## Beta-Thalassemia Intermedia

Patients with β-thalassemia intermedia (β-TI) show clinical pictures of intermediate severity between the thalassemia minor and the transfusion-dependent TM patients. In this condition, an affected person has two abnormal genes, causing a moderate to a severe decrease in β-globin production. They may develop symptoms later than those with TM and with milder symptoms. Some patients with β-TI are asymptomatic until they reach adulthood. They are able to maintain Hb levels between 7-9 g/dL; hence, they do not need or occasional blood transfusion. Severe clinical symptoms may appear between the ages of 2 and 6 years. Approximately 5%-10% of patients survive without blood transfusion [3,5]. The wide range in the clinical severity of β-TI and its borderline with TM can be confusing. The dividing line between β-TI and TM is the degree of anemia and the number and frequency of blood transfusions required. The more a patient depends on blood transfusion, the more likely it is to be classified as TM. Although patients do not need regular blood transfusions to survive, their growth and development are retarded [2,3,6,7].

In general, patients with β-TI need blood transfusions to improve their quality of life, but not to survive. Due to ineffective erythropoiesis, severe β-TI transfusion can lead to iron overload and increased intestinal iron absorption. Ineffective erythropoiesis is a term used to describe active erythropoiesis (the formation of RBCs), the increase in immature erythroblast production, the destruction of developmental erythroid cells in the bone marrow, and the decrease in RBC output, which leads to anemia. Treatment of individuals with β-TI is symptomatic. Splenectomy is a related aspect of the treatment.

## *Beta Thalassemia Major*

TM is associated with the most serious clinical changes and life-threatening risk and is characterized by the triad of chronic anemia, ineffective erythropoiesis, and iron overload. The disease manifests in the first two years of life, usually within 3 to 6 months after birth. Affected infants often fail to grow and gain weight (failure to thrive), and gradually become pale and anemic. They show feeding problems, diarrhea, restlessness, recurrent fever and bleeding tendencies, especially epistaxis. Patients are prone to infection, impairment of the immune system, pathological fractures of long bones, and body organs' dysfunction. When children with TM have symptoms, the Hb level may be as low as 3 to 5 g/dL [3,4,7]. The manifestations of TM depend on the severity of the anemia, the patient's age, duration of the clinical symptoms, the timing and frequency of blood transfusion, age of initiation of iron chelation therapy, and splenectomy. To treat hypoxia symptoms, blood transfusion is required in order to normalize Hb level. The aim of transfusion therapy is the correction of anemia, suppression of erythropoiesis, and inhibition of gastrointestinal iron absorption [8-10]. Initiation of the regular transfusion program can maintain a minimum Hb concentration of 9.5 to 10.5 g/dL and a post-transfusion level of 13 to 14 g/dL. Transfusion prevents growth impairment, organ damage, and bone deformities, allowing normal growth and development up to 10 to 12 years, but complications related to iron overload may occur [3,5,8-10]. In TM, an excessive function of the spleen (hypersplenism) can cause splenomegaly, which can aggravate anemia by eliminating healthy red blood cells in the peripheral blood. This event is associated with a decrease in the number of white blood cells (leukopenia), increasing the risk of infection, and decreased platelets production (thrombocytopenia). The normal spleen is an important part of the body's defense system and a blood filter. It also removes old red blood cells from the body's circulation. TM features including oral, maxillofacial, skeletal, hormonal, cardiac, and liver will be described later.

## EPIDEMIOLOGY

Thalassemia is one of the most common genetic diseases in the world. About 3% (~270 million carriers)of the world's populations carry the thalassemia gene, of which 1.5% (80–90 million people) are the carriers of β-thalassemia [2,11-13]. Every year, nearly 9 million women who are carriers of thalassemia become pregnant, and 1.3 million pregnant women are at risk of TM disease [11]. More than 100,000 UK inhabitants with a nonindigenous ethnic background are carriers of β-thalassemia [12], which is consistent with epidemiological data from Germany and Italy. Globally, about 7% of pregnant women carry β- or α-thalassemia [12]. Males and females are equally affected. Thalassemia presents a major public health and social challenges in high-incidence areas. The frequency and type of the disorder vary considerably between geographic areas and populations. Carriers of thalassemia are higher in the Mediterranean, the Middle East, the Indian subcontinent, Southeast Asia, sub-Saharan Africa, the western Pacific, and south China. Reports on the prevalence of α-thalassemia show that up to 5% of the population in these regions have the trait,while 40–60% are carriers. The α-thalassemias are encountered in the majority of Arab countries in frequencies ranging from 1 to 58 % with the highest frequencies reported from Gulf countries

[14]. In Europe: 1–2% of the population has α-thalassemia trait, and 12% may be a carrier. The highest frequency of β-thalassemia is reported in southern Italy, Greece, and Cyprus, with carrier frequency 10% to 15% [11-13]. The prevalence in Arab countries, Turkey, and Iran ranges from 2.5% to 10%. Over 330,000 affected infants worldwide are born each year (83% sickle cell disorders, 17% thalassemias) [12]. Up to 90% of these births occur in low- or middle-income countries, where transfusion is available for a small fraction of those who need it. Unless iron-chelating therapy is provided, most blood transfusion patients in these countries will die from iron overload. According to the Thalassemia International Federation, only 200,000 patients with TM who received regular treatment worldwide are still alive [4].

India is the country with the largest number of children suffering from TM in the world (150,000), and there are nearly 42 million carriers of thalassemia, with an average prevalence of 3–4% [15]. The Middle East and North African (MENA) region exhibits a high number of TM and carriers due to the tradition of a close relative marriage [12-14]. In Iraq,there are 15,000 registered TM/intermedia patients, mainly Kurds [12]. The prevalence of β-thalassemia in the Al-Hassa region, Saudi Arabia, is 3.4% [16]. In the United Arab Emirates (UAE), the estimated carriers of β- and α-thalassemia are 8.5% and 49%, respectively [17]. In Europe and the United States, the prevalence of thalassemia has increased due to immigrants from endemic countries and intermarriages between different races. Hence, thalassemia has become a disease of international concern [11]. In the United States, thalassemia occurs mainly among Italians, Greeks, and blacks. The incidence of mild α-thalassemia is much greater than that of β-thalassemia.

## CONSANGUINITY

Consanguineous marriage is a deeply rooted social and cultural trend among people in the Middle East, West Asia, and North Africa. It is estimated that one billion people in the world live in communities that prefer close marriage, accounting for 20% to 50% of all marriages [18,19]. The marriage rate among relatives in many Arab countries is the highest in the world. Factors that play a crucial role in the preference of consanguineous marriages are maintenance of family structure and property, ease of marital arrangements, and financial advantages [19-21]. The consanguinity marriage of Iraqis, Jordanians, Saudis, and UAE is between 50 and 60%, Yemenis 44%, and Egyptians and Palestinians 40%. Among the Arab population, there are 25–60% relative marriages, and the rate of first-cousin marriages is 25 to 30% or higher (Fig. **2**). In some parts of Saudi Arabia, intermarriage between close relatives is as high as 80% [22]. Higher congenital malformations in the offspring of consanguineous parents' marriages compared with the figures for the general population have been reported [19-21]. Consanguineous unions, particularly first cousins, have an increased risk of autosomal recessive disorders in children because they share 12.5% of their genetic material. The risk of birth defects in first-cousin marriages is estimated to be 2–2.5 times the general population rate [20].

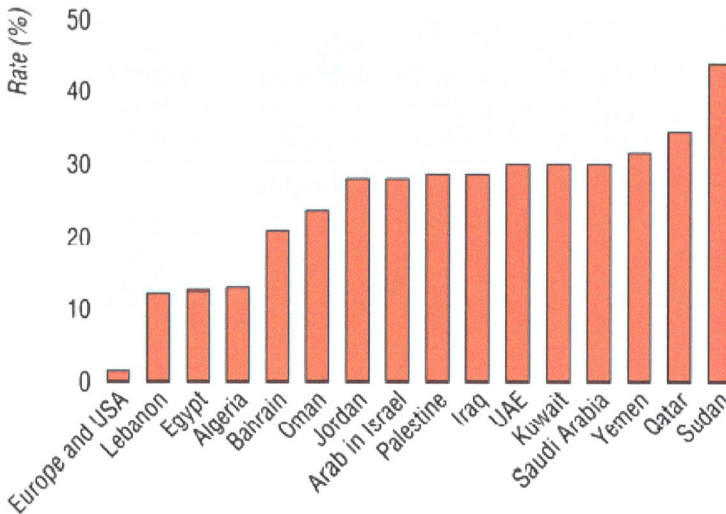

**Fig. (2).** Percentages of average marriages between first cousins among Arabs. [Courtesy of Dr. Lihadh Al-Gazali, BMJ 2006; 333:831-4 [20].

## HEREDITARY TRANSMISSION

Thalassemia is inherited in an autosomal recessive manner. However, inheritance can be very complicated because multiple genes affect the production of Hb. Dominant inheritance has also been reported. Autosomal recessive transmission occurs when an individual inherits the abnormal gene for the same trait from both parents to develop the condition. If a person receives one normal gene and one gene for the disease, the person will become a carrier of the disease, but usually does not show any symptoms. If both parents are carriers of the defective genes, the risk of their children being affected is 25%, and the risk of becoming carriers of the disease is 50% and a 25% chance to not have the condition and not be a carrier (Fig. **3**). With autosomal dominant inheritance, a person only needs to inherit one copy of the abnormal gene in order to develop the disease.

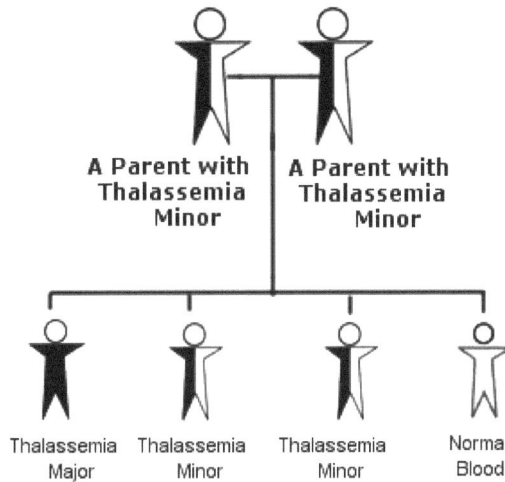

**Fig. (3).** Thalassemia inheritance pattern.

## PATHOPHYSIOLOGY

The pathophysiology of α thalassemia is different from the pathophysiology of β thalassemia. The lack of α-globulin chains will result in a relative excess of β-globulin chains, and the lack of β-globulin chains will result in an excess of α-chains. In β-thalassemia minor, the production of α-chain continues at a near-normal rate. Alpha thalassemia intermedia (HbH disease) causes microcytic anemia, hemolysis, and splenomegaly. In β-thalassemia major or β-intermedia, hemolysis of peripheral RBCs, ineffective erythropoiesis, and reduced Hb synthesis can lead to anemia. The thalassemia anemia stimulates the hematopoietic stem cells in the bone marrow to produce more erythrocytes through erythropoietin, but the produced RBCs are abnormal. Erythropoietin is a hormone mainly secreted by the kidneys, which stimulates erythropoiesis in the bone marrow in response to cellular hypoxia. The main consequence of ineffective erythropoiesis is increased iron absorption and the accumulation of iron in the tissues. Over time, large amounts of ineffective erythropoiesis in the bone marrow cavity of the skull and ribs can lead to bone hypertrophy and expansion by 25–30 times [3]. Ineffective erythropoiesis is the main feature of TM, which leads to the following events: hypertrophy and expansion of the erythroid marrow cavity, impaired bone growth, thinning of the mandibular cortex, increased bone resorption, bone deformation, and increased bone fragility [1-3,5,6,8]. The bone marrow of patients with β-thalassemia contains five to six times the number of erythroid precursors in healthy individuals.

Osteopenia or osteoporosis is characterized by decreased mineralization and can reduce the bone formation sites [1-3,8]. Osteopenia is a precursor to osteoporosis. Osteoporosis is characterized by low bone mass and disruption of bone architecture, resulting in reduced bone strength and increased risk of fractures. The pathogenesis of TM-induced osteoporosis is multifactorial. Genetic and acquired factors play a role in the demineralization of bones in thalassemia. Endocrine complications including hypothyroidism, hypoparathyroidism, diabetes mellitus, and mainly hypogonadism are considered as major causes of osteopenia/osteoporosis in TM. The iron deposits in the bone impair osteoid maturation and inhibit mineralization, leading to focal osteomalacia. The mechanism by which iron overload interferes in osteoid maturation and mineralization includes the incorporation of iron into hydroxyapatite crystals, which affects the growth of crystals and reduces bone metabolism. Severe osteoporosis can cause skeletal abnormalities, fractures, spinal deformities, nerve compression, and growth failure.

Iron overload (hemosiderosis) is associated with increased morbidity in transfusion-dependent patients. It occurs as a result of severe chronic hemolysis of erythrocytes, regular blood transfusions, and the increased absorption of dietary iron in response to the severe anemia and ineffective erythropoiesis. In hemolysis of RBCs, serum bilirubin levels increase (hyperbilirubinemia). Iron overload progressively develops general problems mainly in the heart (cardiomyopathy), liver fibrosis and cirrhosis, endocrinopathy (gonad, thyroid, parathyroid, pituitary, pancreas, and adrenal glands), hypersplenism, venous thrombosis, osteoporosis, growth retardation, and failure of sexual maturation [5-10].

## CLINICAL DIAGNOSIS

Most people with characteristics of thalassemia were identified accidentally, in which a complete blood count showed mild microcytic anemia. Microcytic anemia can be caused by iron deficiency, thalassemia, lead poisoning, or anemia of chronic disease. The diagnosis of thalassemia is based on the anemia phenotype, family history, and relevant laboratory tests. Patients are usually diagnosed through newborn screening programs to determine the presence or absence of Hb. The medical history of patients with thalassemia varies greatly, depending on the type of thalassemia and the severity of the underlying defect. Children who are usually suspected of having thalassemia in unexplained mild microcytic hypochromic anemia, are those being treated for possible iron deficiency anemia and are unresponsive. Clinical presentation of TM usually occurs between 6 and 24 months of life. Both α- or β-thalassemia carriers present with microcytic hypochromic

RBCs with or without anemia, which requires a differential diagnosis to exclude iron-deficiency anemia. After ferritin measurement, family history and ethnicity may provide useful information for the laboratory diagnosis of thalassemia. The physical examination of thalassemia includes the tissue response to decreased oxygen delivery. The first manifestation of TM is an inactive infant with poor growth and development, anemia, and jaundice. Progressive features include tachypnea, scleral icterus, hepatosplenomegaly, bony changes, susceptibility to infection, and other signs and symptoms of anemia. In most cases of mild thalassemia, there are no physical abnormalities. In severe thalassemia, findings are quite remarkable. Typical signs and symptoms of anemia include fatigue, weakness, shortness of breath, irregular heartbeats, chest pain, dizziness, pale or yellowish skin, pale mucous membranes, cold hands and feet, headaches. If left untreated, severe anemia can lead to serious and even life-threatening complications. In TM, hypersplenism can aggravate anemia by eliminating healthy red blood cells in the peripheral blood. This event is associated with a decrease in the number of white blood cells (leukopenia), increasing the risk of infection, and decreased platelets' production(thrombocytopenia). The normal spleen is an important part of the body's defense system and a blood filter. It also removes old red blood cells from the body's circulation.

## LABORATORY TESTING

Both α- or β-thalassemia carriers (heterozygotes) present with microcytic hypochromic RBCs with or without anemia. This requires a differential diagnosis to exclude iron-deficient anemia. Family history and ethnicity may provide useful information in approaching the laboratory diagnosis of thalassemias. The hematological parameters including red cell indices and morphology, followed by separation and measurement of Hb fractions are the basis for the identification of thalassemia carrier [23].

## PRENATAL TESTING

Tests can be performed before the baby is born to find out if he or she has thalassemia and determine its severity. Tests used to diagnose thalassemia in fetuses include Chorionic villus sampling usually done around the 11th week of pregnancy. Amniocentesis is usually performed around the 16th week of pregnancy. Prenatal diagnosis through DNA analysis is now available for many high-risk populations.

## HEMATOLOGICAL TESTING

Blood testing involves analysis of the size, shape, color, and number of RBCs; it is called a complete blood count (CBC). The Hb is also analyzed to determine how much and which types of Hb are present. Standard hematological tests for thalassemia patients include the assessment of mean corpuscular hemoglobin (MCH: average mass of Hb per RBC in a sample of blood), mean corpuscular volume (MCV: average volume of RBC in the blood), and serum ferritin level. Ferritin is a protein in the body's cells that stores iron; mainly found in the liver, spleen, and bone marrow. The concentration of ferritin varies with age and gender. Males have higher values than females. Normal serum ferritin levels for men ranging from 20 to 330 ng/mL and for women are 12 to 300 ng/mL. Serum ferritin is an important tool for evaluating iron stores in the body and monitoring the response to iron chelation therapy. Low ferritin values provide absolute evidence of iron deficiency anemia. Raised levels often indicate iron overload, but they are not specific. Ferritin can be measured using immunoassays; *e.g.*, ELISA [9,10,23]. Iron overload is defined as the serum ferritin levels≥ 1000 ng/L.The basic hematological parameters for the identification of thalassemia carriers include RBC indices and morphology, and measurement of Hb fractions [23].To differentiate iron deficiency anemia from thalassemia in children, the Mentzer index in which MCV, in fL (femtoliters or μm3) is divided by the RBC count  (RBC in millions per microLiter). The ratio in iron deficiency anemia is usually greater than 13, whereas in thalassemia less than 13. A ratio of 13 would be considered uncertain.

Carriers of β-TI or TM have relatively high RBC counts, while MCV and MCH are significantly reduced. They have less severe RBC morphologic changes than the affected individuals [3,9]. The erythrocytes are microcytic, hypochromic, and poikilocytes (Fig. **1**). The number of erythroblasts is related to the degree of anemia and ineffective erythropoiesis, which markedly increased after splenectomy. The Hb level of TM patients is usually reduced to <7g/dL compared with a normal range of 12–17 g/dL depending on gender. The mean MCV ranges between 50 and 70 fL/RBC counts compared to 80–98 fL/RBC counts in a normal range. The average MCH concentration is between 12 and 20 picograms (pg)/cell, while the normal value is 27–32 pg. β-TI is characterized by Hb level between 7 and 10 g/dL, MCV 50–80fL and MCH 16–24 pg. Thalassemia minor also shows some reduction in the MCV and MCH, and RBC morphologic changes with greater Hb level compared to TM and β-TI [3,4,23]. The most widely used cutoff values of MCV and MCH for indicating thalassemia are 79 fL and 27 pg, respectively. Hb test is performed by using electrophoresis and/or high-performance liquid chromatography.

# IRON DEPOSITION TESTING

Liver iron concentration and serum ferritin have been used to monitor iron overload. Serum ferritin greater than 2500 ng/mL or liver iron concentration greater than 15 mg/g dry weight is associated with an increased risk of serious complications and mortality. The liver is the major site of iron overload, containing 70% or more of body iron content. Iron concentration in liver biopsy is highly correlated with the body iron accumulation and basic standard for evaluating iron overload [3,8-10]. However, this is an invasive technique with the possibility of complications. Magnetic resonance imaging (MRI) has been adopted to evaluate iron accumulation in the liver and heart and used as a guide for chelation therapy. It is a non-invasive and reliable method of assessing iron overload. The Myocardial T2*(transverse magnetization) value obtained from MRI is inversely related to tissue iron level. MRI T2* values less than 20 ms (millisecond) indicate myocardial iron overload, and less than 10 ms indicate severe cardiac iron overload. The Magnetic susceptometry method measures the paramagnetic of the liver, which is proportional to the liver iron concentration [10]. Liver biopsy is still used to evaluate liver fibrosis, cirrhosis, or cancer, which may be possible complications in patients with liver iron overload.

# GENETIC TESTING

The introduction of molecular genetic testing helps to detect gene deletions and mutations. Thalassemia mutation test is used to detect the changes in the HbA1 and HbA2 genes of α-thalassemia and the changes in the HbB gene of β-thalassemia, which causes the disease. The test can also be used to provide counseling for the carriers or affected individuals whose offspring are at risk of having the disease, and to monitor pregnancy complications. Molecular analysis is not required to confirm the diagnosis of β-carrier, but it is necessary to confirm the α-thalassemia carrier status. It is also essential to predict severe transfusion-dependent and intermediate-to-mild non-transfusion-dependent cases. DNA analysis is also the only reliable way of diagnosing carriers who have only one of four α-genes deleted or mutated and who have normal Hb and RBCs in the basic blood tests. Especially in α-thalassemia, it is important to know whether a person with α-thalassemia features has two mutant genes on one chromosome or one mutant gene on each chromosome. Other state-of-the-art techniques for DNA analysis are using mass spectrometry or protein sequencing. The continuous reduction in the cost of DNA analysis may lead to its application as a step in the screening process.

Diagnosis of thalassemia and other genetic disorders in the fetus can be made as early as 10–11 weeks of pregnancy using procedures such as amniocentesis (amniotic fluid test) and chorionic villi sampling by removing a tiny piece of the placenta [3,4]. The fetal DNA can be tested with a needle, and a sample of amniotic fluid is drawn from the sac surrounding the fetus, umbilical cord blood, diagnosis and recording of caries is when a lesion in a pit *in-vitro* fertilization technique, *i.e.*, pre-implantation genetic diagnosis (PGD), is used to identify genetic defects in embryos. The procedure involves retrieving mature eggs and fertilizing them with sperm in a dish in a laboratory. Only those without genetic defects are implanted into the uterus. This test enables affected parents to give birth to healthy babies.

## SUBJECTS AND METHODS

Dental and orofacial features of TM was evaluated on 54 Jordanian subjects, 31 males and 23 females aged 5.5 to 18.3 (mean $11.6 \pm 3.2$) years. A thalassemia-free matched by age and gender served as a control group. Family histories revealed that 41% of the patients were the offspring of first-cousin marriage, 32% of second-cousin marriages, and 27% of distantly related or unrelated parents. The average number of siblings per family was 6.1. One-third (31%) of siblings had TM. Clinical, radiographic, and odontometric examinations were carried out to assess changes caused by this disorder. The subjects were examined for oro-maxillofacial features, dental caries, oral hygiene and periodontal status, tooth crown size, dental arch dimensions, dental development, and physical growth. The ethical approval of the study was obtained from the Research Committee of the Jordan University of Science and Technology, and the parental consent of all participants.

### Dental Caries

The sample was divided into four age groups: 6-7, 8-9, 12-14, and 15-18 years old. Teeth were examined for dental caries using plane mouth mirror and sickle-shaped dental probe under standard operating illumination. Before the examination, the teeth were gently dried by compressed air. Dental caries were determined and expressed by dmft (decayed, missing, filled, teeth) for primary teeth and DMFT for permanent teeth, according to the WHO criteria. A tooth is recorded as sound if there is no evidence of treated or untreated clinical caries. A tooth with white spots or stained pits or fissures in the enamel that catch the explorer but not have detectably softened floor is considered sound. The criterion for the diagnosis and recording of caries is when a lesion in a pit/fissure, or on a smooth tooth surface, has a detectably softened floor, undermined enamel, or softened wall. A tooth with a temporary filling is included in this category. On proximal surfaces, the explorer has entered the lesion. All questionable lesions are regarded as sound. The rules for determining deft or DMFT scores include:

- No tooth counted more than once. It is either decayed, missing, filled, or sound. Restoration with recurrent decay is counted decayed.
- Teeth lost due decayed or teeth badly decayed is counted missing.
- A tooth that has several restorations is counted as one 'F' tooth.
- Only, carious cavities are considered as 'D', the initial lesions (white spots. stained fissures, *etc.*) are not considered as 'D'.

The Student's t-test was used to determine the statistical differences between the average dmft and DMFT between males and females and between the test group and the control group [24]. The level of significance chosen was $P< 0.05$.

The Silness-Löe Plaque Index is used to assess oral hygiene. The plaque accumulation on the surface of the six indexing teeth [12, 16, 24, 32, 36, 44] was evaluated using a mouth mirror and explorer. Each of the four surfaces of the teeth (buccal, lingual, mesial, and distal) is given a score from 0 to 3 as follows:

- Score 0: No plaque.
- Score 1: A film of plaque adhering to the free gingival margin and adjacent areas of the tooth. Dental plaque can only be seen *in situ* after applying a disclosing solution or using a probe on the surface of the tooth.
- Score 2: Moderate accumulation of soft deposits in the gingival pocket and/or on the tooth and gingival margin, which can be seen with the naked eye.
- Score 3: Abundance of soft matter in the gingival pocket and/or on the tooth and gingival margin.

## Periodontal Status

Simplified Oral Hygiene Index (OHI-S) is composed of the combined Debris Index and Calculus index, which was used to evaluate oral hygiene status. The OHI-S on the six surfaces of the indexing tooth was checked. Calculus deposit was determined by placing a dental explorer into the distal gingival crevice and drawing it subgingivally to the mesial contact area. TheOHI‑S criteria(index and grade) are as follows:

- Score 0 (zero): No soft debris/calculus.
- Score 1: (up to 1.2); soft debris/supragingival calculus cover less than one-third of the tooth surface.
- Score 2: (1.3–3.0); soft debris/supragingival calculus cover one-third of the tooth surface.
- Score 3: (3.1–6.0); soft debris/supragingival calculus cover more than two-thirds of the tooth surface or a continuous heavy band of subgingival calculus around the cervical portion of the tooth (Fig. **4**). Periodontal status and oral hygiene were assessed using a plane mouth mirror, sickle-shaped explorer, and periodontal probe with William's markings (1-3,5,7,8-10 mm). The periodontal pocket (probing pocket depth, PPD) was assessed by measuring the distance from the free gingival margin to the bottom of the sulcus [25] (Fig. **5**).

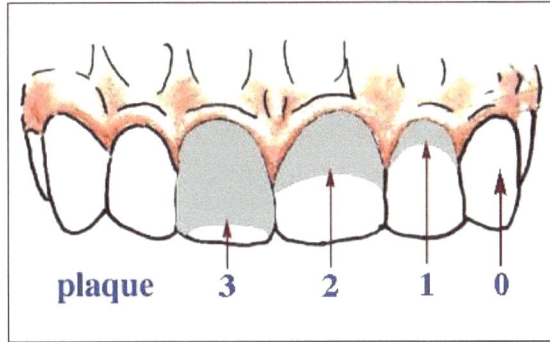

**Fig. (4).** Criteria for scoring plaque.

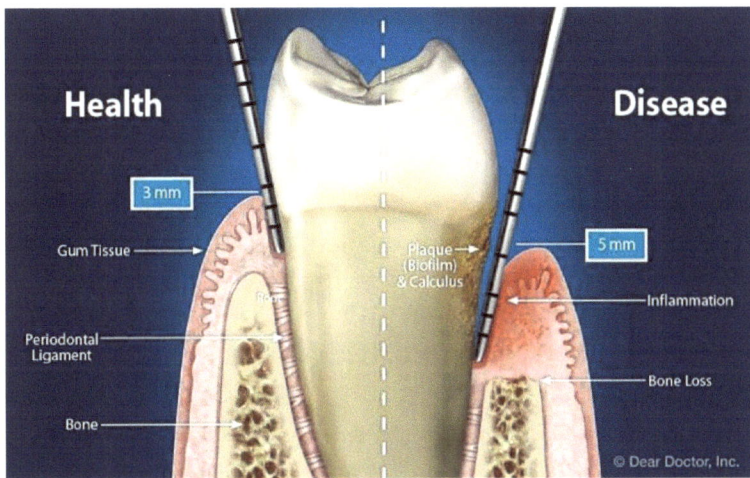

**Fig. (5).** Periodontal probe (Williams probe, 1 to 10 mm marking) to assess periodontal pocket-depth. Note the inflamed gingiva. [By Dr. Mario A. Vilardi. From: https://www.deardoctor.com/articles/understanding-periodontal-pockets]. Google Images.

Gingivitis was assessed for the six index teeth using the criterion of the gingival index (GI) of Löe and Silness (1963). The index teeth examined were the maxillary right first molar (# 16), maxillary right central incisor (# 11), maxillary left first molar (# 26), mandibular left first molar (# 46), mandibular left central incisor (# 41), and the mandibular right first molar (# 36). The gingival index to score gingival health is as follows:

- Score 0: Normal gingiva.
- Score 1: Mild inflammation—a slight change in color, slight edema. No bleeding on probing.

- Score 2: Moderate inflammation—redness, edema, glazing. Bleeding on probing.
- Score 3: Severe inflammation— marked redness and edema, ulceration. Spontaneous bleeding. A numerical score of the GI as follows: 0.1–1.0 mild gingivitis, 1.1–2.0 moderate gingivitis, 2.1–3.0 severe gingivitis.

## Tooth Crown Measurement

Mesiodistal crown diameter (MD); also known as tooth size, tooth crown size, or tooth width, has been used in human evolution, biology, anthropology, forensics, and other fields. In clinical dentistry, MD provides a wealth of information, including the interrelation between the MD and the arch alignment. The sample consisted of 45 TM patients, 25 male and 20 female, aged between 7.3 to 18.3 years, with a mean age (±SD) of $11.2 \pm 3.6$ years [26]. The control group consisted of 198 healthy subjects from the same community, tested in a previously validated study [27]. The MD and buccolingual (BL) crown diameters were measured on the maxillary and mandibular permanent teeth [26-28]. Alginate impressions were taken using suitable perforated trays for the upper and lower dental arches, which immediately cast in the dental stone. Teeth selected for measurements only when are completely erupted, free from abrasion or caries or restored, and of normal crown shape. The MD is recorded from the first molar on one side to the corresponding tooth on the contralateral side by measuring the greatest distance between proximal surfaces (contact points) of the crown. Measurements were performed by using a fine tips electronic digital sliding caliper reading to the nearest 0.01 mm. The sexual dimorphism in tooth crown size is expressed by the percentage of the crown diameters of males over the females, as follows: 100 (male mean MD divided by the female mean MD minus 1). Except for the third molars, the BL crown diameter was measured for the maxillary and mandibular teeth. Using the digital caliber placed parallel to the long axis of the tooth, measurement was taken for the greatest distance between the buccal/facial (vestibular) and lingual surfaces of the tooth crown (Fig. **6b**). Analysis of variance (ANOVA) and Student t-test were used to assess the differences between parameters.

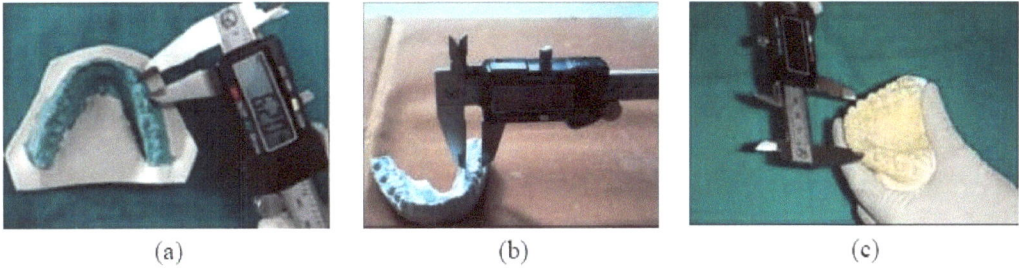

**Fig. (6)**. **(a)** Measure mesiodistal width. **(b)** Measure buccolingual width. **(c)** Measure dental arch dimensions (length and width).

## Dental Arch Dimensions

The shape and size of dental arches provide a wealth of information for dentistry, biology, anthropometry, and other disciplines. Maxillary and mandibular dental arches'dimensions were measured on dental casts using the digital caliper (Fig. **6c**). Measurements include the arch depth, anterior and posterior arch lengths, inter incisor, inter canine, inter premolar, intermolar arch widths (Fig. **7a** and **b**). *Arch depth*: The distance from the line connecting the distal surface of the first molars to the midpoint between the central incisors.

• *Anterior Arch Length*: The distance between the mesial contact point of the central incisor and the distal contact point of the canine.

• *Posterior Arch Length*: The distance between the mesial contact point of the canine and the distal contact of the second premolar.

• *Interincisor Width*: The distance between the distal contact point of the lateral incisor on one side to the distal contact point of the contralateral tooth.

• *Intercanine Width*: The distance between the cusp tip of the canine on one side to the cusp tip of the contralateral canine.

• *Interpremolar Width*: The distance between the buccal cusp tip of the second premolar on one side to the buccal cusp tip of the contralateral second premolar.

• *Intermolar Width*: The distance between the mesiobuccal cusp tip of the first molar on one side to the mesiobuccal cusp tip of the contralateral first molar.

Arch perimeter (circumference) is measured using a brass wire of 0.5-mm diameter contoured along the line of occlusion from the distal aspect of the first molar passing around the arch on the center of the contact area to lie over the incisal edges of the anterior teeth and to the distal aspect of the contralateral first molar[29]. Differences between test and control groups were statistically analyzed.

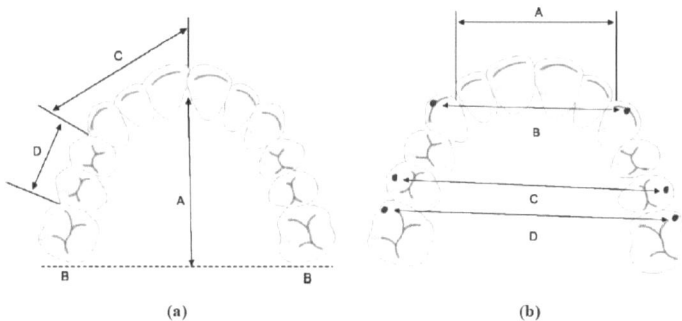

(a)     (b)

**Fig. (7).** **(a)** Measurements of dental arch **lengths** (A – arch depth; B – arch perimeter; C –anterior arch length; D – posterior arch length). **(b)** Measurements of dental arch **widths** (A – inter-incisorwidth; B – intercanine width; C – inter-premolar width; D – intermolar width).

## Tooth Size Ratio

The correct MD relationship between the maxillary and mandibular teeth is very important to achieve a balanced occlusion during the final stages of orthodontic treatment. For proper occlusion, the tooth size must be consistent with the arch size, and the sum of the widths of mandibular teeth must be smaller than the sum of the widths of the maxillary teeth. In order to determine the discrepancy between the size of maxillary and mandibular teeth, and their impact on interarch relationship, Bolton'sindex of Anterior and Total tooth size ratio is used as follows:

$$\text{Anterior ratio} = \frac{\text{Sum of MD of mandibular six anterior teeth (33 to 43)}}{\text{Sum of MD of maxillary six anterior teeth (13 to 23)}} \times 100$$

$$\text{Overall ratio} = \frac{\text{Sum of MD of mandibular 12 teeth (36 to 46)}}{\text{Sum of MD of maxillary 12 teeth (16 to 26)}} \times 100$$

## Mandibular Linear and Angular Measurements

Linear and angular measurements of the mandible were obtained from tracing the panoramic radiographs on overlying acetate papers. The measurements were carried out as shown in Fig. (8).

● Maximum ramus width: The distance between the most anterior and posterior points on the mandibular ramus.

● Ramus length (height): The distance between the highest point of the condylar head (process) to the lowest point on the posterior border of the mandible.

● Minimumramus width: The distance between the deepest point on the anterior and posterior borders of the ramus.

● Intercondylar distance: The distance between the highest point of the head of the right and left condyles.

● Gonial angle: The angle between the one-line tangent to the lower border of the mandible and another line tangent to the distal border of the ascending ramus and the condyle [25].

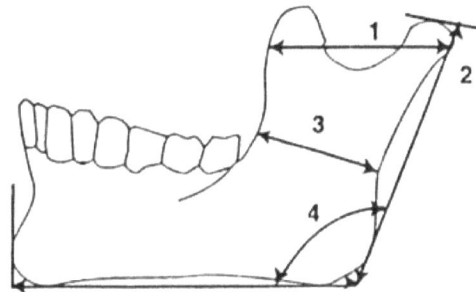

**Fig. (8).** Schematic drawing showing dimension measurements of the mandible after tracing panoramic radiographs and using the digital caliper.1– Maximum ramus width. 2–Ramus length (height). 3– The smallest (narrowest points) ramus width. 4 –Gonial angle.

## Physical Growth

The 54 TM patients were assessed for height, weight, and BMI, by age group, with the respective values from the standard Jordanian growth chart. The patients were divided into six groups from 6–7 to 16–18 years old. Height was measured using a wall-mounted stadiometer. The patient stood upright, took off his shoes and heavy clothes. Bodyweight was measured on a digital scale to the nearest 0.1 kg. The patient's physical growth pattern was compared with a standard growth chart for school-age children. The body mass index (BMI) was calculated as body weight in kilograms divided by the square of the height in meters (kg/m$^2$), which indicates the nutritional status of a person. Low body mass index (underweight) of <18.5. Normal weight = 18.5–24.9. Overweight = 25–29.9.  Obesity = 30 or greater.

## Dental Development and Chronological Age

The development of human teeth is a continuous process, starting from the sixth week in the uterus until about six months after the birth of the primary dentition, and from the sixteenth week in the uterus until the late adolescence period of the permanent dentition. No other organs of the human body takes so long to reach its ultimate development as the dentition. The maxillary primary central incisor begins calcification (3-4 months) in utero, followed by the first molars, lateral incisors, canines, and second molars. The radiograph of the 30-weeks old fetus showed that the 3/5 crown of the mandibular anterior teeth is complete. At birth, about 60% to 80% of the crowns of the primary incisors are completed, and about 30% of the canine crown is fully formed. The permanent central incisors begin calcification 3 to 4 months after birth and the second premolar and second molar from 2 to 3 years.

The tooth development and eruption process go through a series of well-defined stages that are controlled by the local, systemic, environmental, and genetic factors. Changes in tooth development may cause abnormalities in the number, structure, form (size or shape), and color of teeth. Dental age (DA) assessment is important in pediatric dentistry, orthodontics, medicine, biology, forensics, legal action, asylum seekers, criminal, and birth certificates [30]. The development of teeth is relatively independent of the maturity of other systems and can act as a marker of aging. Several biological indices have been used to determine the developmental stage relative to chronological age (CA), including sexual maturity, somatic maturity, and DA. Skeletal age estimation involves correlating biological age (or physiological age) with CA (the length of time a person has been alive). A significant difference was found between skeletal age and DA. This discrepancy arises because biological age varies between individuals, while CA is measured by time. Biological age is a function of genetics, environmental factors, hormone levels nutrition, and gender.

DA is the chronology of tooth development from the embryological origin of the tooth bud to the progressive sequence until a complete eruption in the oral cavity. Radiography of permanent teeth is used to determine the stage of tooth development and provides valuable and reliable indicators for the DA and CA indexes [30,31]. Another dental method used to determine CA is to visualize the stage of tooth eruption clinically. Using tooth eruption to determine the CA is unreliable because many factors (for example lack of space, ankylosis, and early or delayed exfoliation of primary teeth) can alter the eruption of permanent successors. The most widely accepted method of estimating tooth development is to measure the degree of calcification of permanent teeth using panoramic radiographs, as described by Demirjian *et al.* [31]. This method evaluates tooth development from the first appearance of calcification points (stage A) to the closure of the root apex (stage H) (Fig. **9**). In this method, the seven left mandibular permanent teeth (second molar to central incisor) of each participant are rated on an eight-stage scale of dental maturity. The method of determining the tooth maturity, DA, and DA of TM patients has been described elsewhere [30].

## Stages of Tooth Development

Stage A: Beginning of calcification. Calcified points at the superior level of the crypt as an inverted cone or cones without fusions.

Stage B: Fusions of calcified points form one or more cusps, which unite to give a regularly outlined occlusal surface 1/3$^{rd}$ crown completed.

Stage C: Crown half-formed and dentinal deposition is occurred.

Stage D: The crown 2/3$^{rd}$ or completely formed and the beginning of root formation.

Stage E: The root 2/3$^{rd}$ root is completed and an initial formation of the radicular bifurcation.

Stage F: The apex ends are a funnel shape; the root length is equal to or greater than the crown height.

Stage G: Root is completed and the apical end is partially open.

Stage H: Apical foramen closed.

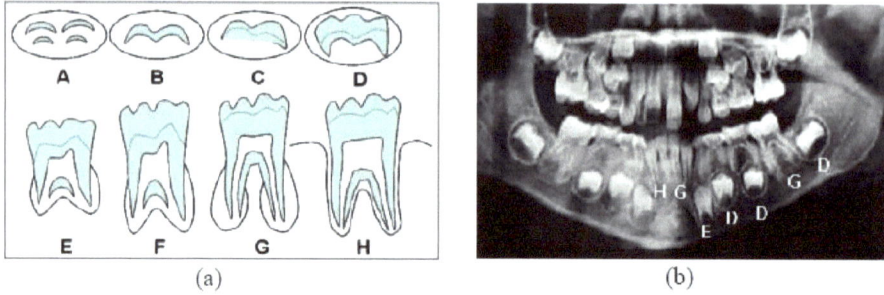

(a)                                                                    (b)

**Fig. (9).** Stages of tooth development. **(a)** Schematic drawings of the eight stages of crown-root formation of the mandibular molar according to Demirjian *et al.* method. **(b)** Panoramic radiograph showing stages of tooth development of a 7-year-old child. Note: Tooth development in girls is usually ahead of the boys and there is a wide variation in tooth development between individuals.

**Plate 1** shows the teeth development stages, DA, and the corresponding CA of normal children, which can be used as a reference for thalassemia patients and other applications.

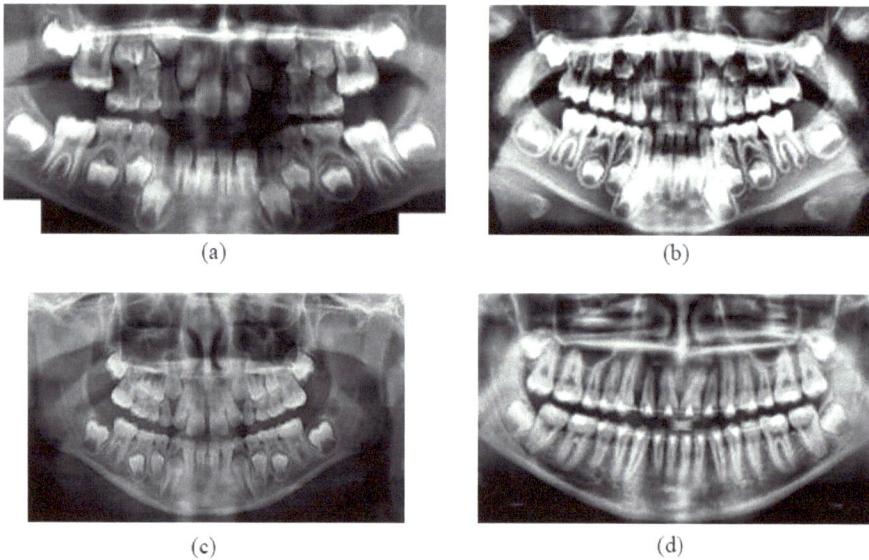

(a)                                                                    (b)

(c)                                                                    (d)

**Plate (1).** Panoramic radiographs show the stages of tooth development and DA in normal children based on the formation of crowns and roots. **(a)** A 6-year-old child: The first permanent molars have emerged above the CEJ of the second primary molars, and the root apical end is partially opened. **(b)** An 8-year-old child: The first permanent molars and central incisors have fully erupted, and crown 2/3rd of the second permanent molars is formed. **(c)** A $9^{1/2}$ aged child: The crown of the second permanent molar is fully formed, with initial roots formation. **(d)** A 12-year-old-child: Teeth have erupted near to the line of occlusion, and 2/3$^{rd}$ of the third molar crown is completed.

# RESULTS

## Oro-maxillofacial Features

In TM, the oro-maxillofacial features are the result of bony changes due to ineffective erythropoiesis, and the formation of erythroid mass with bone expansion. These changes are characterized by bossing forehead and cheekbone, saddle nose, maxillary protrusion, flaring of the maxillary anterior teeth, increased overjet and open bite, lip incompetence, and malocclusion [32,33]. Of the 54 TM patients, 33% had an almost normal appearance (Grade 1, Plate **2a**), 26% had mild changes (Grade 2, Plate **2b**), and 16.7% had a 'chipmunk face' (Grade 3, Plate **2c**).

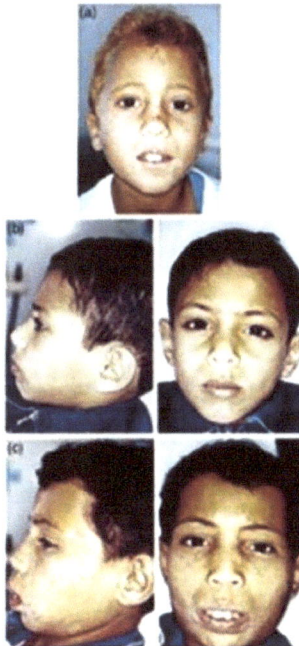

**Plate 2.** Grades of maxillofacial deformities in TM children.

**Grade 1a**: Slight depression of the nasal bridge and minor maxillary overgrowth.

**Grade 2b**: The frontal and cheek (malar) bones are slightly prominent; the upper jaw is barely enlarging; the bridge of the nose is depressed and the eyelids are swollen.

**Grade 3c**: Forehead (frontal bone) bossing; prominent cheekbones (malar bones), saddle nose; gross maxillary overgrowth; protrusive maxillary anterior teeth; lip incompetence; excessive overjet; giving a "chipmunk" appearance, and a tendency of eye slanting and flaring of nose alae [32].

Table 1. Prevalence of orofacial TM features in different population groups.

| TM sample | Jordanian[25] | Iranian [36] | Indian [37] |
|---|---|---|---|
| **Sample size, % and (n)** | **54** | **119** | **72** |
| Frontal bone bossing | 61.1 (33) | -- | -- |
| Saddle nose | 59.2 (32) | 34.0 (40) | 56.9 (41) |
| Lip incompetence | 51.8 (28) | 47.9 (57) | 80.6 (58) |
| Discolored teeth | 44.4 (24) | -- | -- |
| Dental and jaw pain | 40.7 (22) | -- | -- |
| Pallor oral mucosa | 38.9 (21) | 26.9 (32) | 22.2 (16) |
| Headache | 29.6 (16) | -- | -- |
| Increased overjet | 25.9 (14) | -- | -- |
| Maxillary protrusion | 24.9 (13) | 49.7 (149) | 60.5 (72) |
| Chipmunk faces | 16.7 (9) | 34.7 (104) | -- |
| Nasal airway problem | 16.7 (9) | -- | -- |
| Lower lip paresthesia | 13.0 (7) | -- | -- |
| Parotid gland enlargement | 5.6 (3) | -- | -- |

## Dental Caries

The mean dmft and DMFT values and their components of the 54 TM patients assigned to the age groups (Table **2**). Females had higher caries experience than males: dmft 7.31 vs 6.54 for the 6–7-year age group and DMFT 6.67 *vs* 5.83 for the 12–18-year-old group. Because the differences did not reach the significance level ($P<0.05$), the data for males and females were combined (Table **2**). No significant difference was found between the dmft and DMFT values. The main contributor to dmft and DMFT scores is tooth decay, which accounts for 95.2% of the total dmft and 92.7% of the total DMFT value. Between the ages of 6 and 9, the average dmft for thalassemia patients was 5.82. For 12–14 years old, the DMFT value was 6.57 and 5.95 for 15–18 years old. Compared with the healthy control group, the incidence of caries in TM patients was significantly higher. Overall, the average DMFT of 15-year-old patients was 6.26, while the DMFT of the control group is 4.84 ($P<0.001$). Only 17.4% of TM children aged 6–9, and 21.4% of those aged 15 years have no caries[24]. Importantly, 36.2% of 6–9-year-old patients and 45.8% of 12–18-year-old patients had 5 or more carious teeth. The average plaque score of TM patients in the 6–11-year-old group was $1.57 \pm 0.44$ ($\pm$SD), and the $1.74 \pm 0.57$ for 12–18-year-old. The corresponding scores of the healthy control group were $1.43 \pm 0.63$ and $1.67 \pm 0.68$, respectively (Table **3**). No significant differences between age groups and gender were found. The overall mean plaque score of the 54 TM patients was $1.67 \pm 0.52$.

**Table 2. Caries experience in primary teeth (dmft) and permanent teeth (DMFT) and their components in the TM age group [24].**

| Age Group | Primary Teeth | | Permanent Teeth | |
|---|---|---|---|---|
| (years) | 6-7 | 8-9 | 12-14 | 15-18 |
| Decayed | 6.59 | 4.29 | 6.09 | 5.33 |
| Missing | 0.25 | 0.18 | 0.26 | 0.35 |
| Filled | 0.08 | 0.25 | 0.22 | 0.27 |
| Total dmft/DMFT | 6.92 | 4.72 | 6.57 | 5.95 |
| (SD) | (4.54) | (3.86) | (4.28) | (3.74) |

**Table 3. Oral hygiene and periodontal status of TM patients and control group assessed by plaque index (PI) and gingival index (GI) [25].**

| Age Group (mean ± SD) (years) | Thalassemic Group (mean ± SD) | | Control Group | |
|---|---|---|---|---|
| | PI | GI | PI | GI |
| 6–11(n = 23) | $1.57 \pm 0.44$ | $1.30 \pm 0.49$ | $1.43 \pm 0.63$ | $1.24 \pm 0.40$ |
| 12–18 (n = 31) | $1.74 \pm 0.57$ | $1.56 \pm 0.69$ | $1.67 \pm 0.68$ | $1.48 \pm 0.61$ |

## Periodontal Status

Compared with the control group, TM patients had higher OHI-S and GI scores (Table **3**). The mean OHI⁻S score of the patients was $2.12 \pm 0.64$, while the OHI⁻S score of the control group was $1.73 \pm 0.69$. The difference is statistically significant ($P<0.01$). Only 5.5% showed no visible plaque deposits. About two-thirds (61%) of the patients had moderate accumulation of soft deposits within the gingival pocket (score 2) and 33.4% had a thin plaque film deposit (score 1). The dental calculus deposition rate in the test group was 32.5%, while the control group was 21.8%. The GI score showed that 49.2% of patients had mild gingivitis, 34.7% had moderate gingivitis, and 8.3% had severe gingivitis. Only 7.8% showed no sign of gingivitis, compared with 25.2% in the control group. In the test group and control group, the GI scores were significantly higher in older ages than those of the young ($P<0.025$). Among these patients, 16.7% had a gingival sulcus depth of 3 mm, 6.1% had a pocket depth of 4–5 mm, and 1.9% had a pocket depth of $\geq 6$ mm. The mean periodontal pocket depth (PPD) of the  patients was $2.7 \pm 1.4$ mm, while that of the control group was $2.3 \pm 1.2$ mm [25]. The periodontal pocket represents the transition from the normal gingival sulcus to the pathologic periodontal pocket. A tendency of higher frequency and mean of periodontal disease in TM group compared with control group did not reach the significant level of $P<0.05$.

## Tooth and Mucosal Discoloration

Due to chronic jaundice in TM, the incorporation of pigment bilirubin (a degradation product of Hb) in the dentinal tubules during tooth formation results in yellow discoloration of teeth [34]. The discoloration of teeth and oral mucosa of thalassemia patients (Fig. **10**) was 44.4% and 38.9%, respectively.

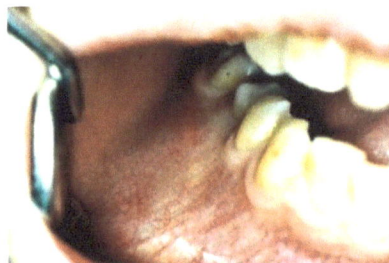

**Fig. (10).** Pallor oral mucosa and yellowish dental discoloration in TM [25].

## Tooth Crown Size and Tooth Size Ratio

In males and females, there is no significant difference between the MD values of the teeth on the left and right sides of the dental arch. The maximum difference is 2.25% of the average measured value. All mean values of MD in TM males and females were smaller than the control group, and 20 of the 24 comparisons were statistically significant, ranging from $P<0.05$ to $P<0.001$ [26]. Males of thalassemia have a greater MD than females, and the differences range from 0.12 mm for the mandibular second premolars to 0.48 mm for the maxillary first molars. The weighted difference is 0.28 mm on average. The MD of the thalassemia group was reduced by 0.31 mm on average compared with the control group. The cumulative MD of the maxillary and mandibular teeth in the thalassemia group (sexes pooled) was 92.0 mm and 84.7 mm, respectively. The corresponding values for the control were 95.6 mm and 88.4 mm, respectively. The difference between the test group  and control group was statistically significant ($P<0.001$). The relative variability in MD estimated by the coefficient of variation (CV=SD/ mean x 100) showed that the lateral incisors exhibited the greatest variability in both thalassemia and control groups (CV=7.6%) whilst the first molars displayed the least variable teeth (CV=5.3%).

In the TM group, the cumulative BL dimensions of the maxillary and mandibular of males were 120.9 mm and 110.3 mm, respectively. The corresponding values for females are 116.3 mm and 105.7 mm [28]. As for MD, the BL value of the thalassemia group was significantly lower than that of the control group. The degree of symmetry between pairs of antimeric teeth (using the Pearson coefficient of correlation), shows that the r-value of  MD is between 0.61 and 0.80, while the r-value of BL is between 0.60 and 0.86. Sexual dimorphism percentages in the MD of thalassemia and control groups were similar (3.7% *vs.* 3.6%). The order of ranking sexual dimorphism by the morphological classes is canines (5.4%), molars (4.1%),  incisors (3.3%), and premolars (2.9%). The mandibular central incisor is the least dimorphic (1.7%), while the mandibular canines (5.9%) displayed the greatest dimorphism in thedentition[27,28]. The anterior and the overall percentages of tooth-size ratios (sexes pooled) in the thalassemia group were 79.1 and 92.0, respectively. The corresponding ratios of the control group were 79.4 and 92.4, respectively. There was no significant difference in the anterior and overall ratios between sexes and between the thalassemia group and the control group. The anterior and overall ratios in both the thalassemia and control groups were significantly larger ($P<0.001$ and $P<0.05$, respectively) than the Bolton ratios for the ideal occlusion.

## Dental Arch Dimensions

The dental arch size plays an important role in obtaining a functionally stable occlusion, well-aligned teeth, proper arch form, and proper overjet and overbite. They are of particular interest for orthodontists to understand occlusion changes during the stages of development and in the diagnosis, planning, and orthodontic treatment. The measurement results showed that, compared with the control group, the length of the maxillary arch and the mandibular arch of the TM group were reduced by 2.59 mm and 2.55 mm, respectively. No significant difference was found in the arch length on the left and right sides of the dental arch. Compared with the control group, the anterior arch length of the test group was 1.76 mm shorter in the maxilla and 1.63 mm shorter in the mandible. The mean maxillary and mandibular arch depths were shorter by 3.21 and 2.63 mm relative to the controls. Compared with the control group, the arch width of thalassemia patients was significantly reduced by 1.33 to 1.90 mm in the maxilla and 1.37 to 1.77 mm in the mandible. The thalassemia group had the largest reduction in the interincisal width of the two arches compared with the control group ($P<0.001$). In the maxilla, the reduction of the interincisal width was 1.82 mm and 1.70 mm in the mandible. The mean maxillary and mandibular arch perimeters were reduced by 3.91 and 3.44 mm in the thalassemic group compared with the controls [29]. The difference in arch parameters between the test group and the control group was highly significant ($P<0.001$).

## Occlusion and Cephalometric Analysis

Cephalometric measurements of thalassemia and the control group were performed to assess the relationship between teeth, jaws, and facial skeleton in the three age groups of 5 to 18 years of age. Measurements show that almost all TM patients have a Class II skeletal relationship, maxillary protrusion, and a relatively short mandible (Fig. **11**). The hypertrophy of the maxilla leads to the increased overjet, spacing, and protruding anterior teeth, accompanied by different degrees of malocclusion (Fig. **12**). In 25.9% of TM patients, an increase in overjet was found. The average ANB angle of TM patients was significantly larger than that of the control group ($P<0.05$). Patients showed a reduced anterior cranial base length (S–N) compared with the controls ($P<0.05$). The mandibular length (Ar–Gn) of the patients was lower than that of the controls (88.6 ± 7.9 mm *vs.* 98.8 ± 6.9 mm, $P<0.001$), and the biggest difference was in the young age group (7.5 years old). On the vertical plane, the total facial height (Na–Me) was significantly less than that of the controls (105.4 ± 5.9 mm *versus* 112.8 ± 4.8, *P<0.01*). Thalassemia patients had reduced posterior facial heights (Ar–Go and S–Go) averaged 35.3 ±

4.9 mm and 61.1 ± 5.3 mm, respectively. The corresponding heights in controls were 40.1 ± 3.7 mm and 66.5 ± 3.9 mm. These differences were statistically significant (*P<0.01*). The maxilla appeared prominent (3.3 mm in males and 5.1 mm in females) due to a reduced cranial base length (Ar–S) and a short mandible (Ar–P) [35].

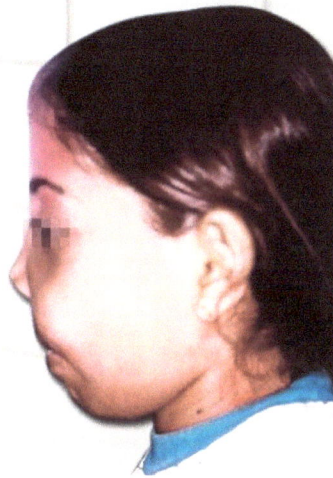

**Fig. (11).** A 14-year-old girl showing typical facial features of TM. Note: prominent frontal and check bosses, saddle nose, and mandibular atrophy [29].

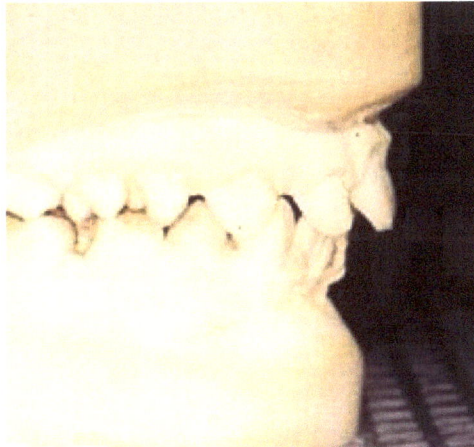

**Fig. (12).** Dental cast of TM patient showing maxillary protrusion, flaring of the maxillary anterior teeth, spacing of teeth, increased overjet, and malocclusion [25].

## Dental Development

Tooth development assessment showed that 79.5% of TM patients had delayed dental development (representing the DA) compared with CA. It was found that the average tooth development delay was $1.12 \pm 0.58$ ($\pm$SD) years for males and $0.81 \pm 0.53$ years for females, with a total average of 0.97 years ($P<0.001$, df=38) [30]. As compared with males, females had a more advanced formation of dentition. An example of DA relative to the CA is shown in Fig. (**13**). The association between DA and CA is stronger than that between DA and body growth ($r = 0.87$ *vs.* 0.58) [30].

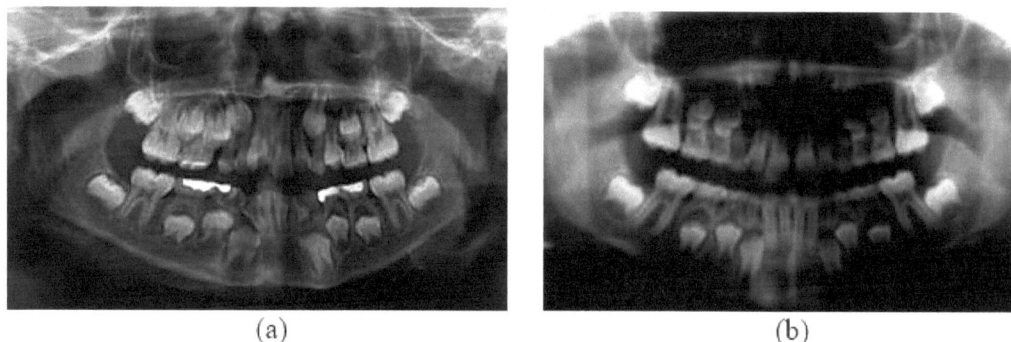

(a)                                                          (b)

**Fig. (13). (a)** A panoramic view of a 9.8-year-old boy with TM showed that tooth development was delayed by 1.1 years compared with the tooth development of an 8.7-year-old healthy boy **(b)**.

## Physical Growth

The weight, height, and BMI of TM patients by age were compared with the corresponding values in the standard Jordanian growth chart. Growth retardation ($<10^{th}$ percentile for height and weight) was present in 75.9% of the TM patients. Height less than the $3^{rd}$ percentile was noted in 41.9% of males and 34.8% of females. Growth retardation is more pronounced in patients over 10 years of age. The patient's body mass index (BMI) was 14.1 to 18.7 ($kg/m^2$), $16.3 \pm 1.8$ $kg/m^2$ for males and $16.9 \pm 2.3$ $kg/m^2$ for females. The average value on the standard chart is $18.5 \pm 2.8$ $kg/m^2$. In patients under 10 years of age, BMI is less than 21.6%, while in patients over 10 years of age, BMI is less than 10% [30].

## Mandibular Measurements

Linear and angular radiographic measurements of the mandible in TM patients revealed a significant reduction in the ramus length of average 3.2 mm and width 1.8 mm, compared with the control group. The intercondylar distance in the TM group was reduced by 6.9 mm. The average gonial angle of the thalassemia group (127.3°) was significantly greater than that of the controls [25].

Table 4. Prevalence of TM radiographical features.

| TM Sample | Jordanian [25] | Indian [38] |
|---|---|---|
| **Sample Size, % and (n)** | **33*/ 48*** | **50** |
| Thickened frontal bone * | 66.7 (22) | -- |
| Thinned mandibular cortex** | 64.6 (31) | -- |
| Indiscernible mandibular canal borders | 62.5 (30) | 74 (37) |
| Maxillary sinus hypoplasia* | 42.4 (14) | 36 (18) |
| Faint lamina dura** | 39.6 (19) | 26 (13) |
| Enlarged marrow spaces ** | 37.5 (18) | 50 (25) |
| Widened diploic spaces* | 36.4 (12) | -- |
| Short spiky roots ** | 33.3 (16) | 56 (28) |
| Taurodontism** | 24.8 (12) | 82 (41) |
| "Hair-on-end" calvarium* | 6.1 (2) | -- |

* Lateral radiographs, ** Panoramic radiographs.

## Radiographic Features

Cephalometric and panoramic radiographs have been used to assess dental, and craniofacial changes in TM patients. The results are listed in Table **2** and shown in Figs. (**14-20**). In most patients, there was thickening of the frontal bone (Fig. **14**) and thinning of the inferior border of the mandible (mandibular cortex) (Figs. **14** and **15**). Faint or absence of mandibular canal borders in 62.5% of the patients' radiographs (Figs. **15–17**). Maxillary sinus in 42.4% of the patients' radiographs (Fig. **14**). More than one-third of the patients have a faint lamina dura, enlarged bone marrow spaces, and widened diploic spaces in the frontal bone (Figs. **14–16**). Normal lamina dura *(arrows)* appears as a thin radiopaque layer of compact bone that lies adjacent to the periodontal ligament (Fig. **18**). Short and spiky roots of the mandibular molars observed in 33.3% of the patients' radiographs (Figs. **15** and **16**). Taurodont molars in one-fourth of the patients' radiographs (The alveolar bone displays generalized rarefaction due to enlarged marrow spaces and altered trabecular pattern, characterized by the apparent coarsening of some trabeculae and the blurring or disappearance of others producing "chicken-wire" appearance (Fig. **19**). The appearance hair-on-end skull is a relatively uncommon radiographic finding. It is an alternating opaque trabecula and diploic radiolucent marrow oriented perpendicular to the inner and outer tables of the skull, giving appearance of long, thin vertical striations in a radial pattern (Fig. **20**). Panoramic radiograph of the anatomical landmarks of a normal subject is shown in Fig. (**21**).

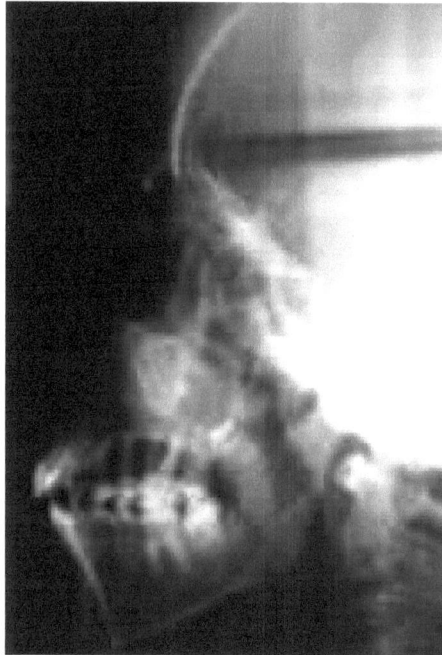

**Fig. (14).** Cephalometric skull radiograph of a 15-year-old boy with TM showed thickening of the frontal bone, prominent premaxilla, small maxillary sinus, and enlarged diploic spaces (the the cancellous bone between the inner and outer tables of the calvarium was expanded) [25].

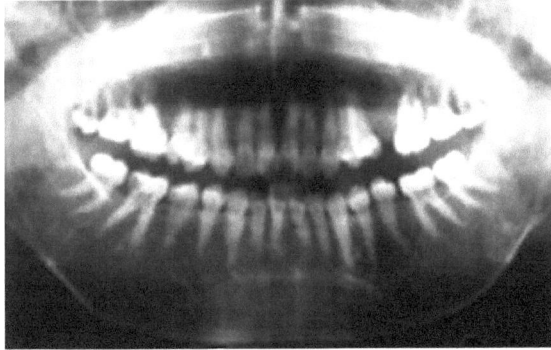

**Fig. (15).** Panoramic radiograph of TM patient showed thinning of the mandibular inferior cortex, indiscernible borders of the mandibular canal, enlarged bone marrow spaces, absence of trabeculae, short and spiky roots of the mandibular molars, and faint lamina dura [33].

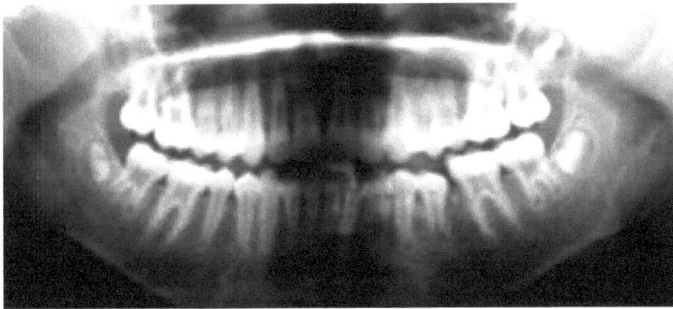

**Fig. (16).** Panoramic radiograph showing taurodont molars and short spiky roots.

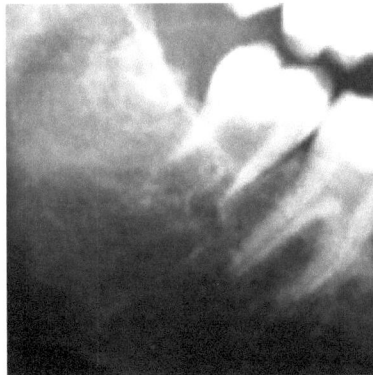

**Fig. (17).** Close radiographic image of TM patient disclosing absence of borders of the mandibular alveolar canal and taurodont molars.

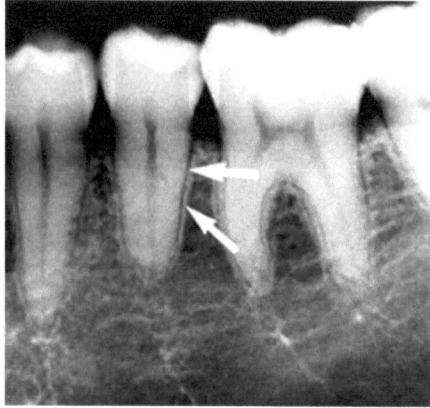

**Fig. (18)**. The normal lamina dura (arrows) appears as a thin radiopaque layer of the dense bone surrounding the tooth socket. It is thicker than the thin radiopaque rods (trabeculae). The absence of trabeculae suggests the presence of diseases such as thalassemia and sickle cell anemia.

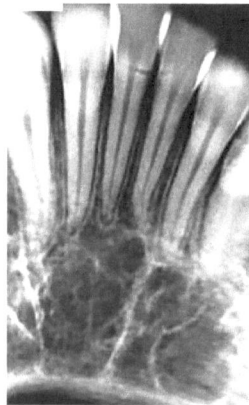

**Fig. (19)**. Periapical radiograph of TM patient showing large bone marrow spaces and sparse course trabeculae; producing "chicken-wire" appearance in the alveolar bone proper [Source: https://www.slideshare.net/vahid199212/systemic-diseases-manifested-in-the-jaws].

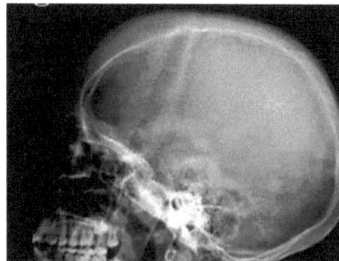

**Fig. (20)**. Lateral skull radiograph of TM patient showing 'hair-on-end" appearance in a skull radiograph. It is seen in the diploic spaces of the skull radiograph and appearing like long, thin vertical striations similar to standing hair that associated with hemolytic anemias such as thalassemia and sickle cell disease [Google Images].

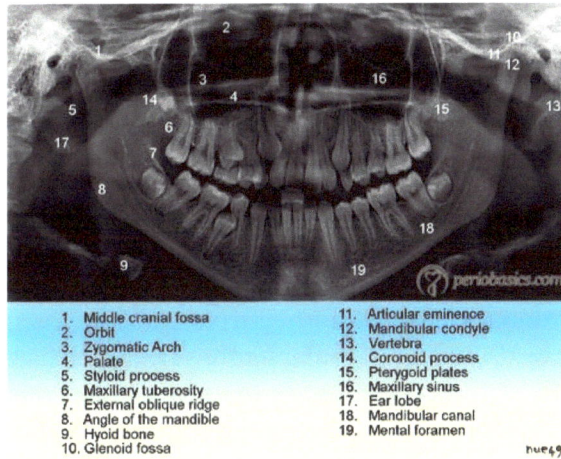

**Fig. (21)**. Panoramic radiograph shows normal anatomical landmarks of a normal subject. It views a large area of the maxilla and mandible on a single film and depicts numerous anatomic structures outside of the jaws. Note the normal thickness of the mandibular inferior cortex, superior and inferior borders of the mandibular canal, and maxillary sinus landmarks. [Source:https://www.pinterest.de/pin/331155378840585487/].

## DISCUSSION

Thalassemia is an autosomal recessive inheritance of chronic hemolytic anemia, which is caused by insufficient or lack of synthesis of α- or β-globin chains due to mutations in the corresponding genes. The first suspicion that a patient has a Hb disorder is seen in a full blood count test. Because iron deficiency anemia shows a very similar picture, it's important to rule it out before diagnosing thalassemia, which can be diagnosed once the iron deficiency has been treated. In the presence of an abnormal full blood count and normal iron status, more specialized tests are required to confirm the diagnosis of thalassemia. Among thalassemia types, TM is associated with the most severe clinical changes and life-threatening risks. In the progressive course of illness, the condition is characterized by iron overload, cardiomyopathy, infection, liver fibrosis and cirrhosis, endocrinopathy, hypersplenism, osteoporosis, growth retardation, and failure of sexual maturation, with typical signs and symptoms of anemia [1-3,5]. TM leads to serious medical, social, psychological, and economic problems for patients and their families as well as budget and care burden for the public health services. The primary treatment for TM involves regular blood transfusions at 3-4 week intervals. This is necessary to maintain Hb at normal levels and treat the anemia. Successful treatment depends on early diagnosis, regular blood transfusion, iron chelation, infection control, and treatment facilities. If given appropriate treatments, many patients in developed countries can survive to the fourth or fifth decade of life [13, 39].

Advances in diagnostic tools and medical care continue to improve the life expectancy and quality of life of TM patients.The way in which the family and the patient come to cope with the disease and its treatment will have a critical effect on the patient's survival and wellbeing. Today, the classic clinical picture of TM is primarily seen in countries with insufficient resources to provide affected individuals with treatment (*e.g.*, regular blood transfusions and iron-chelation therapy). Allogeneic hematopoietic stem cell transplantation was until very recently, the only permanent curative option available for patients suffering from transfusion-dependent β-thalassemia. Gene therapy, by autologous transplantation of genetically modified hematopoietic stem cells, currently represents a novel therapeutic promise byre-establishing effective hemoglobin production. Patients may be rendered transfusion- and chelation-independent and evade the immunological complications that normally accompany allogeneic hematopoietic stem cell transplantation.

## LITERATURE REVIEW

### Dental and Orofacial Features

The distinctive orofacial features in patients with TM are due to intense hyperplasia of the bone marrow and expansion of the marrow cavity in response to severe hemolytic anemia, chronic hypoxia, and ineffective erythropoiesis.TM oro-maxillofacial changes include:

- bossing of the frontal bone;
- prominence of the malar bone;
- thinning mandibular inferior cortex;
- indiscernible mandibular canal borders;
- altered trabecular pattern;
- obliterated maxillary sinuses;
- enlarged marrow spaces;
- widened diploic spaces;
- reduced dental arches dimensions;
- premaxilla protrusion;
- flaring and spacing of the maxillary anterior teeth;
- teeth discoloration;
- pale oral mucosa;
- lip incompetence;
- faint lamina dura;
- short spiky roots;
- increased overjet and open bite;
- malocclusion (Tables **1** and **2**).

These abnormalities become more prono-unced with age. Generally, if blood transfusion therapy is started in early childhood and the Hb level is maintained at 9–10 g/dL, the orofacial features of TM patients will become minimal.

In TM patients, the impedance of the maxillary antrum pneumatization leads to a smaller antrum, which may be due to the compression caused by the expansion of the maxillofacial bones and hypertrophy of the marrow cavities. The thinning of the mandibular inferior cortex and the reduction or loss of the inferior alveolar canal boundary may be the sequelae of bone marrow expansion, increased bone resorption/erosion, and decreased bone mineral density. The thin mandibular cortex is associated with osteoporosis [40,41]. Overgrowth of bone marrow in the maxillofacial bones may cause lateral displacement of the orbit and eye slanting

(Plate **2c**). Lack of lip seal may be due to maxillary protrusion and proclined maxillary anterior teeth. This leads to mouth breathing and dryness, which exacerbates dental caries and periodontal disease. The pallor of the oral mucosa may arise from the chronic anemia underline the TM. Flaring of nose alae (Plate **2**) is adaptive to air/oxygen hunger caused by the hypoxia of anemia. Dental pain in TM patients may due to pulpal blood vascular infarction/thrombosis, which leads to pulpal necrosis. Painful swelling of the parotid glands and reduced salivary secretions can be a result of iron deposition. Thalassemic patients experience dental and jaw pain, transitory headaches, and lip paresthesia [25, 33].

The orofacial deformities in Jordanian TM patients aged $11.6 \pm 3.2$ years (Plate **1**) is comparable to those earlier reported by Logothetis *et al.*, [42] on Greek TM patients (mean age $10 \pm 4$) where 32% had a normal appearance, 23% had mild maxillary overgrowth, and 14% had "rodent-like faces." The prevalence of orofacial TM features of Jordanians and other population groups is shown in Table **2**. Elangovanetal. [37] reported that among 72 Indian TM patients (aged 6 to 18 years), 41.7% had a rodent face, 56.9% saddle nose, 80.6% lack of lip seal, 22.2% pale oral mucosa, 18.1% anterior open bite. Radiographic examinations of 50 Indian TM patients showed 82% taurodontism, 56% spiky short roots, 26% faint lamina dura, 50% large bone marrow spaces, 36% obliterated maxillary sinuses, 26% absence of inferior mandibular canal [38] (Table **3**). In a study on 60 Thaiβ-thalassemia major, Wisetsin [43] found that 73% of the patients had thin mandibular cortex, 63% had thickening of the frontal bone and parietal bones, 8% had "hair-on-end" calvarium, and 5% absence of maxillary sinus. Abd - ulla and Husen [44] who examined 50 Iraqi TM patients reported that 68% had enlarged bone marrow spaces, 60% tooth discoloration, 48% Class II malocclusion, 28% saddle nose, 28% thin lamina dura, 24% spiky roots, and 16% taurodont molars (sexes pooled). A study on 300 Iranian TM patients, Salehi *et al.* [45] found that 67% had saddle noses, 49% had a maxillary protrusion, 41% had mucosal discoloration, 34% had rodent face, 20% had teeth spacing, and 8% had an open bite. In addition to genetic and ethnic influences, the significant differences in the frequency of TM manifestations between different studies can also be explained by the severity of the disease, course of treatment, sample size, patients' age, and the diagnostic standards used.

**Mandibular Inferior Cortex**

Since the change in the width (thickness) of the mandibular inferior cortex is an important feature of TM and related osteoporosis, it needs to be reviewed. Reynolds (1965) reported that the mandibular cortex is considered thin when its width is measured 4 mm or lesser compared to a normal thickness of about 6 mm [46]. With the use of a computer-aided system and the presence of sensitive equipment, the normal cortex width is found lesser than that earlier reported by Reynolds. My literature review of 14 recent studies on healthy and osteoporotic patients (mean age 46 ± 18) shows that the normal mandibular cortex width varies from 3.2 mm [47] to 6.5 mm [48], with an average of 4.98 ± 0.87 mm. The threshold for osteoporosis ranges from 2.9 mm to 4.5 mm (mean 3.34 ± 0.75 mm). The thickness of the mandibular inferior cortex detected on dental panoramic radiographs can help identify osteoporosis [49,50]. A Polish study of elderly patients with osteoporosis showed that the width of the cortex (2.9 mm) was highest at the age of 30-39, and then gradually decreases [51]. Hattab [25] reported that two-thirds (64.6%) of TM patient shave a thinning of the mandibular cortex (<3.3 mm), usually accompanied by a faint or absence of the inferior mandibular canal borders (Figs. **15** and **18**).In a contradiction with the well-documented cortical bone thinning in TM, a study said "Thirty-five patients (70%) were between 4.5 mm and 6 mm" [52], the results should interpreting with caution.

## Dental Caries

Although dental caries is a multifactorial disease with several causative factors, there is evidence for a genetic component in the etiology of this disease.The high incidence of dental caries in TM patients are documented in different population groups [24,44,53,54]. De Mattia *et al.* [54] studied the prevalence of dental caries in 60 Italian TM patients. They reported a DMFTscore of 5.12, where only 8% were caries-free.In a study on 15-year-old Jordanian TM children, Hattab *et al.* showed that the DMFTof the TM patients was 6.26 and that of healthy controls was 4.84 [24]. The World Health Organization (WHO) has set DMFT to be very high above 5.6 [55]. The reasons for caries risk in patients with TM can be attributed to poor oral hygiene [24,26,44], reduced salivary flow rate [24,56,57], lower level of salivary immunoglobulin [57,58] high count of salivary streptococcus mutans [58], and neglected dental care.

## Periodontal Disease

Periodontal disease includes a variety of inflammatory conditions that damaging the tooth-supporting structure.TM patients have a higher incidence of periodontal disease compared with the control group [25,33,45,53,59]. Kaplan *et al.* (1964) reported that 32% of the American TM patients had gingivitis and 10% had periodontal pockets [60]. Pedullà *et al.* [53] found that Italian TM patients aged 22 to 55 years had a significantly higher incidence of gingivitis and pocket depth than patients with β-thalassemia intermedia and healthy controls. In addition to poor oral hygiene; reduced saliva flow, mouthbreathing, malocclusion, nutritional deficiencies, infection, and impaired immune system are the triggers for the development of periodontal disease in thalassemia patients. A recent study showed that salivary aspartate aminotransferase and alanine aminotransferase levels in TM patients were much higher than those in healthy controls [61]. These enzymes are potential markers of periodontal disease activity.

## Oral Tissues Discoloration

The gingiva of TM patients exhibit brown to black pigmentation due to iron deposition, parallel to the accumulation of iron in the liver [62]. One explanation for the discoloration of the gingiva is that the excessive breakdown of abnormal circulating RBCs leads to the release of Hb and its by-products. Pallor oral mucosa was found in 38.9% of Jordanian thalassemic patients (Table **2**). A study on 36 Indian TM patients showed that 69% had gingival pigmentation and 78% had pallor oral mucosa [59]. About 30% of 119 Iranian TM patients had gingival discoloration and 27% had oral mucosa pale [36]. Kaplan *et al.* [60] reported a frequent occurrence of pale oral mucosal in TM patients, while De Mattia *et al.*[54] found only three cases of the 60 patients had pale atrophic mucosa. Pale of the oral mucosa in TM is a characteristic of underlying chronic anemia, in which the amount of oxidative Hb is reduced and the serum bilirubin level is increased. Hyperbilirubinemia in TM is secondary to RBCs hemolysis and ineffective erythropoiesis, resulting in yellowing of teeth and skin. The tooth discoloration in TM may shift to brownish discoloration with age [34]. Increased oral Candida albicans colonization was noted in the TM patients [61,63], particularly in splenectomized patients.

## Tooth Crown Size and Tooth Size Ratio

The correct tooth size relationship between the maxillary and mandibular teeth is essential to achieve the optimal functional occlusion, proper interdigitation, and proper overjet, and overbite. Without a correct match of the MD of the maxillary and mandibular teeth, good occlusion cannot be obtained. Different tooth sizes have been associated with different ethnic groups, so it is logical to expect that differences in tooth widths can directly affect tooth width ratios. The most common malocclusion is caused by large tooth size compared to the size of the supporting bone; this creates a tooth-size arch-size discrepancy and dental crowding. The MD of the thalassemia group was reduced by an average of 0.31 mm compared with the control group. The dental sexual dimorphism, obtained by MD measurement, of thalassemic  and  control groups, were similar (3.7% *vs.* 3.6%), calculated as follows: [(Xm /Xf)-1] ×100, where Xm = mean male tooth dimension, Xf = mean female tooth dimension. In both thalassemia and controls, canines displayed the most sexual dimorphic teeth [27, 28]. Root length of the permanent teeth was also used for the determination of dental sexual dimorphism. In forensic dentistry, MD measurement of posterior teeth (the greatest sexual dimorphism) is a valuable tool for determining gender type. Teeth have a highly mineralized structure that allows them to resist postmortem decomposition.

The indices for a correct occlusion, extrapolated from Bolton's studies, are the Anterior Bolton Index (ABI)and the Overall Bolton Index (OBI). The ABI = 77.2 % (74.5–80.4%) and the OBI = 91.3% (87.5–94.8%). An overall ratio of more than 91.3% means that the mandibular teeth are bigger than normal, while a ratio smaller than 91.3% would mean the mandibular teeth are smaller than normal. An anterior analysis follows the same principle. Having a different ratio than normal is referred to as Bolton Discrepancy. A standard deviation of more than 2 yields a significant discrepancy. The anterior and overall percentage tooth-size ratios (sexes pooled) in the thalassemia group were 79.1 and 92.0, respectively. Both ratios are significantly larger than Bolton ratios.

The variations in the tooth size between individuals and different populations reflect a complex interaction between genetic, racial, and environmental factors [64,65]. The genetic contribution to tooth crown size is over 80%. A comparative study between Iraqis, Jordanians, Yemenites, and Caucasians revealed that Jordanians and Iraqis had a larger tooth crown size than the tested populations [27]. Several maternal conditions and gestational variables have an influence on tooth size including diabetes, hypothyroidism, hypertension, birth weight, and length [66,67]. The reduced tooth size may result in a deficiency of the dentoalveolar bone that houses the teeth. Evidence supporting the relationship between reduced tooth size and smaller dental arches has come from studies in patients with chondrodysplasia [68], Down's syndrome [69], oligodontia [70], and cleft lip and palate [71].

**Dental Arches Dimensions**

The size and shape of the dental arch are affected by many factors. These include genetics, environment, pathological entities, and ethnic diversity, as well as local factors such as eruptions; position; and the number of teeth. The difference between tooth crown size and dental arch length can cause crowding of teeth, which is the most common type of malocclusion. Changes in the width, length, depth, and form of the arches will affect the occlusal relationships. The dental arches in patients with TM are shorter and narrower compared with the healthy controls. The mandible is less protruding than the maxilla because the cortex of the mandible is so dense that it cannot expand [29]. Radiographic examination showed a reduction in ramus length and an increase in gonial angle in TM patients compared with the healthy controls [25]. Owing to the lack of studies on changes in the size of the mandible in thalassemia, these findings can not be compared with others. Cephalometric measurements of patients with sickle cell disease revealed a reduction in the ramus length of 1.8 mm and an increased gonial angle of 4.5° compared with the controlgroup [72]. The reduction in dental arch size in TM patients can be a reflection of their general growth retardation and cranial changes [29,32].

## Occlusion and Cephalometric Analysis

An ideal occlusion represents the perfect interdigitation of the upper and lower teeth, which is achieved through proper jaw growth, normal tooth formation and eruption, and simultaneous development of teeth and bones. Skeletal malocclusion in TM patients is caused by a hyperplasia of the bone marrow, bone expansion, and increased bone remodeling of cranial bones. This leads to protruding maxillary anterior teeth, increased overjet, teeth spacing, and inconsistent tooth size and arch length. The frequency and type of malocclusion in TM patients vary considerably among studies determined clinically or radiographically. A clinical study has shown that 55% of Indian patients with TM had Class II malocclusion [73]. Cephalometric analysis of TM patients showed that almost all have Class II dental and/or skeletal malocclusion [35,74,75], manifested by the retrognathic mandible, prognathic maxilla, or combination of both. The protrusion of the maxilla is due to the decrease in the length of the cranial base and the increase in the SNA angle. Adequately blood transfused patients showed lower incidence and severity of malocclusion compared with the low transfused group [75].

## Radiographic Features

Radiographic findings of the teeth and jaw of patients with TM are short and spiky roots, faint lamina dura, taurodontism, large bone marrow spaces, indistinct inferior mandibular canal, and thinning of the mandibular cortex. Kaplan *et al.*, (1964) reported that 86% of their American TM patients had enlarged bone marrow spaces [63]. Their findings are higher than those of Jordanians (37%) [25] and Indians (50%) [38]. The difference may be due to improved disease management, including early diagnosis and initiation of blood transfusion. The incidence of taurodontism

(82%) in Indian TM patients is much higher than that in Jordanians (24.8%) (Table **2**). The differences between the two studies may be due to the differences in the criteria used to identify taurodontism, besides the ethnic variations. Taurodont teeth are more common in the maxilla than the mandible, and the second molar is the most commonly involved tooth. There was no significant difference between males and females in imaging examinations of TM. Nutrient canals in the mandible were observed in 26% of TM patients, compared to 50% in the controls [38].

## Dental Development and Chronological Age

The tooth development and eruption process go through a series of well-defined stages that are controlled by the local, systemic, environmental, and genetic factors. Among the 20,000–25,000 genes in the human genome, about 200 or more genes are directly or indirectly involved in tooth development. Several physiologic growth processes are involved in the progressive development of the teeth including initiation, proliferation, histodifferentiation, morphodifferentiation, apposition, calcification, and eruption. The total time required for an individual tooth to fully develop is quite long, starting from the first appearance of the calcification point to the appearance of the tooth, the completion of mineralization, and eruption into the oral cavity. For the primary teeth, the duration is 2 to 3 years, and for the permanent tooth, the duration is 8 to 12 years except for the third molars. Dental age (DA) is one of the most reliable methods for estimating chronological age (CA). The development and maturation of teeth in TM patients are significantly delayed. The correlation between DA and CA is much stronger than the correlation between DA and body growth [30,31,76-78], because the development of teeth is less affected by environmental factors than physical development. Garn *et al.* [66] found that the delay in dental development is about one-third of the delay in bone development. Greater delay in skeletal maturation than in dental development has been found in children with anemia, hypothyroidism, hypopituitarism, short familial stature, and cerebral palsy [77, 78].

## Growth and Development

Physical growth is a complex process influenced by genetic, hormonal, and environmental factors. Although genes and hormones play an important role in the regulation of body growth, environmental factors can also explain the differences between individuals. Unfavorable environmental factors; such as malnutrition, negative psychology, social status, and pollutants can adversely affect growth. The cause of growth retardation in TM patients is multifactorial including chronic anemia, hypoxia,transfusion-related iron overload, chelation toxicity, malnutrition, racial factors, endocrinopathies (hypothyroidism, hypogonadism, growth hormone), and low socioeconomic status [1-3,5,8]. In different populations, the growth of TM patients is significantly delayed [30,79-83]. Hattab [30] reported that 75.9% of 54 TM children and adolescents in Jordan had retardation in height and weight, which was below the 10th percentile on the standard chart. The growth retardation becomes more pronounced in patients over 10 years of age. Borgna-Pignatti *et al.* [79] reported that among 250 Italian adolescents with TM, 62% of males and 35% of females had short stature. Kattamis *et al.* [80] found that among 405 Greeks with TM, 21.7% of males and 13% of females had growth retardation, with the highest incidence between 15 to 20 years of age. A study of 68 Chinese children in Hong Kong revealed that 75% of TM girls and 62% of boys older than 12 years were below the 3rd percentile of height [81]. Data indicates that TM patients are short, underweight, have a low rate of growth, and decreased BMI [30].

A review of the literature reveals differences in the age at which growth retardation occurs in the TM children. Reports on Italian and Greek patients indicated that slowing of growth was more evident as puberty approached [79,80], while retarded growth in Turkish TM children was found at the age of 8–10 years [82]. A recent study on Indian TM children showed significant growth retardation in height and weight occurs after age 11 years in boys and after age 9 years in girls [83]. Data on Jordanian TM shows that growth retardation worsens after the age of 10 years [30]. Lapatsanis *et al.* [84] observed that half of TM children aged 5–7 years had bone retardation, and after this age bone retardation occurs in almost two-thirds of the cases. It is noted that adherence to modern transfusion regimes and iron chelation protocol reduces the risk for short stature.

## MORBIDITY AND MORTALITY OF TM

The last decades have witnessed advances in understanding the pathophysiology of thalassemia disease and the introduction of novel treatments that improved the clinical outcomes of the disease. Thalassemia-related complications increase the morbidity and mortality of elderly patients, who now live longer than in the past. Complications include anemia, iron overload, infections, cardiomyopathy, pulmonary hypertension, extramedullary hematopoiesis, osteoporosis, thrombosis, splenomegaly, and endocrinopathies [3,5-10]. Iron overload is the main cause of morbidity and mortality related to heart disease, liver and pancreas dysfunction, impaired immune system, endocrinopathy, growth retardation, osteoporosis, and splenomegaly.

Regular blood transfusion is the mainstay of care for people with TM by improving anemia and suppresses ineffective erythropoiesis that leads to compensatory bone marrow expansion and skeletal changes. Blood transfusion can also increase childhood growth and prolong survival. Blood transfusions for children with TM usually begin in the first 2 years of age. Increased gut iron absorption occurs in non-transfused patients as a consequence of increased ineffective erythropoiesis. TM patients who receive irregular blood transfusions usually die before the second or third decade. However, this life-saving therapy is associated with numerous complications "second disease". In treating anemia, the accumulation of iron in the body tissues occurs. Iron overload becomes fatal in the second decade of life if not controlled [9,10,85,86]. The main cause of death is a cardiac failure due to iron overload. Infection is the second most common cause of morbidity and mortality in TM patients, becoming the main cause of death in Western countries [87-89]. Over the years, significant progress has been made in controlling iron-induced heart disease.

The survival and quality of life of patients with β-thalassemia in developed countries have improved markedly in recent decades [39,85,86,89]. Blood transfusion and iron chelation strategies are used to control the disease in the long term and improve the quality of life. In addition, advances in hematopoietic stem cell transplantation technology provide treatment options for certain patients. There is evidence that the survival time of the affected individual who receives regular blood transfusions and appropriate chelation therapy has exceeded 40 years of age [39,85,86]. In developing countries; modest availability of proper medical care, safe and adequate blood transfusions, high therapy cost, and poor compliance to chelation therapy remain major obstacles [12-14]. Early diagnosis and treatment of thalassemia are essential to limit complications because the pathologic process increases with age.

## Iron Overload

In healthy humans there are no controlled mechanisms for the excretion of excess iron, hence body iron is regulated at the sites of absorption, utilization, and recycling. In the physiological state, 1–2 mg of iron is absorbed from food sources daily and the same amount is excreted fecally. Iron overload of body tissues in TM with or without transfusion is fatal if not prevented or adequately treated. For patients who are not receiving transfusions, iron absorption increases several-fold depending on the severity of erythroid expansion [9,10,89]. Regular blood transfusions can double the rate of iron accumulations. Most clinical manifestations of iron loading do not appear until the second decade of life in patients with inadequate chelation. Among patients who received blood transfusions but did not undergo chelation therapy, symptomatic heart disease may appear within 10 years after the initiation of blood transfusion. The burden of transfusion iron overload is related to the frequency, amount, and duration of blood transfusion therapy. Lifelong blood transfusion, chronic hemolysis, and high intestinal absorption of iron can lead to increased iron deposition. This ultimately leads to cardiomyopathy, liver and pancreas dysfunction, and endocrine disorders [3,5,7-9,89]. Other complications of iron overload are hypersplenism, venous thrombosis, osteoporosis, growth retardation, and failure of sexual maturation due to iron loading in the anterior pituitary [8, 9, 86].

Due to the lack of a mechanism for the human body to excrete excess iron, iron overload occurs in patients who are dependent on regular blood transfusion therapy [4,7,9,10]. According to the recommended blood transfusion protocol for TM, 100-200 mL RBCs per kilogram of body weight per year is equivalent to 0.32-0.64 mg iron/kg body weight/day or 116-232 mg/kg/year. If chelation therapy is not given, iron loading rates of patients' weight 20, 35, or 65 kg are averaging 3.4, 6.2, or 11.3 grams per year. The corresponding daily iron loads were 9.4, 16.8, and 30.9 mg, respectively [9]. Hence, unless chelation therapy is provided, blood transfusion therapy will increase the iron load too many times the normal level. Patients with poor blood transfusion can absorb about 3-5 mg/day or more of iron per day through the intestine, which means that an additional 1-2 grams of iron are absorbed every year [3,5,9]. Poorly transfused individuals can absorb around 3–5 mg/day or more of iron through their gut, Hemolysis and chronic hypoxia can further increase intestinal absorption. Paradoxically, despite the massive increase in the body's iron load, excessive iron absorption still exists.

One unit of blood transfusion (420 ml) contains approximately 200–250 mg of iron, and the human body cannot excrete more than 1–2 mg of iron per day [3,89]. Mainly through the shedding of the epithelial cells from the intestine. Patients who receive 25 units per year (every 2 weeks) will accumulate an average of 5 grams of iron without chelation therapy. In addition to the increasing iron absorption from the gastrointestinal tract. Excessive iron is toxic to human cells and may cause severe and irreversible functional damage. Iron overload eventually leads to the following sequelae: hypogonadism, (35–55% of the patients), cardiomyopathy (11.4%–15.1%), liver disease (21%), hypothyroidism (9–11%), diabetes (6–10%), heart failure (6.8%), arrhythmia (5.7%), hypoparathyroidism (4%), human immunodeficiency virus (1.7%) and thrombosis (1.1%) [3, 86, 90, 91].

## Infection

Infection remains one of the major causes of morbidity and mortality in patients with TM. The prevalence of infection in patients with TM varies from 22% to 66% [86-89]. The mechanisms of increased susceptibility to infection in these patients include: (1) impaired chemotaxis and phagocytosis of macrophages and neutrophils, (2) alterations in the T- and B-lymphocytes,(3) decreased the number and activity of natural killer cells, (4) reduced the secretion of immunoglobulin (5) inhibit the function of the complement system [87-89,93,94]. Where infection is suspected, the main reasons to consider are splenectomy; transmission of pathogens by blood transfusion; iron overload; and iron chelation. Splenectomy plays an important role in susceptibility to infections [89,93-95]. The risk of death from infection after splenectomy ranges from 38% to 69% [95-97]. Patients who have undergone splenectomy are at higher risk of massive infection after bacteremia. The most frequent pathogens are *Streptococcus pneumonia, Hemophilus influenza, Klebsiella pneumonia, Neisseria meningitidis, Escherichia coli, and Yersinia enterocolitis* [87,88,93,95]. In the presence of excess iron, many of these organisms increase their virulence. Chronic hepatitis is caused by viral infections that cause hepatitis B and/or hepatitis C.

Overwhelming post-splenectomy sepsis is an emergency and requires immediate antibiotics treatment. Antibiotics include intravenous infusion of Cephalosporin (Cefotaxime, 2 grams every 8 hours or Ceftriaxone, 2 grams every 12 hours) combined with Gentamicin (5–7 mg/kg every 24 hours) or Vancomycin (1–1.5 gram every 12 hours) [96,97]. Children should receive pneumococcal and influenza vaccines after six months of age, and meningococcal vaccination after 2 years of age. Anti-pneumococcal vaccination and prophylactic antibiotics can prevent severe pneumococcal infections in the first 2–4 years after splenectomy. All patients with transfusion-dependent thalassemia should be protected by vaccination against Hepatitis B virus (HBV). If the titer of anti-HBs (hepatitis B surface antigen) decreases, a booster dose of HBV vaccine should be considered [96-99]. Annual serologic testing for Hepatitis and HIV should be performed.

## Cardiac Complications

Cardiac dysfunctions due to chronic anemia and hemosiderosis (myocardial siderosis) are the major causes of death in patients with thalassemia intermedia and TM, leading to morbidity and mortality of 64% to 71% [7,85,88,89]. When the heart is exposed to high circulating iron for a long period of time, it usually deposits 20 grams of iron, which leads to the accumulation of iron in the heart. The myocardial iron overload induces heart failure in patients without chelation as early as the second decade of life. Therefore, cardiac function is monitored annually beginning at 7 or 8 years of age by electrocardiogram, echocardiogram, and recently by cardiac T2* MRI, which can detect preclinical cardiac iron accumulation [102]. The main causes of death are congestive heart failure and fatal cardiac arrhythmias [3,10,85,86]. The new chelation regimens with the adoption of MRI and magnetic susceptometry to evaluate iron overload have contributed significantly to the reduction in cardiac morbidity and mortality in patients with TM. This reduction was obvious after the year 2000 [39,85,104]. Serum ferritin levels are routinely used to identify patients with an increased risk of heart and liver diseases through evaluating the iron store and monitoring the response to iron chelation therapy. Patients with a serum ferritin concentration below 2,500 μg/L have a heart disease-free survival of 91% after 15 years, while patients with a serum ferritin concentration of more than 2500 μg/L have a survival rate of less than 20% after 15 years [5,9,10]. A significant correlation was found between serum ferritin levels and T2* MRI results.

## Endocrine Complications

Endocrine dysfunctions are among the most common complications in TM mostly due to iron overload and suboptimal chelation. Of the hormonal disorders involved are 86% hypogonadism, 23% hypoparathyroidism, and 18% hypothyroidism. Diabetes mellitus ranges from 6 to 30% of patients with TM [105-107]. Although diabetes mellitus is multifactorial, it is attributed to impaired secretion of insulin secondary to chronic pancreatic iron overload. The liver is the main site of iron overload. Liver disease is a common complication of TM caused by hepatitis virus infection and iron accumulated through blood transfusion. Both factors can lead to cirrhosis, which represents a risk factor for hepatocellular carcinoma and the risk of death [92]. For patients with insufficient blood transfusion and chelation therapy, liver disease is a common cause of death after 15 years of age. A close correlation was found between iron deposition in the heart and deposition in endocrine tissues [2,3,9,101]. Iron overload in the pituitary is the main cause of infertility and hypogonadism [89,103,106]. Early administration of iron chelation is effective in preventing endocrine complications with 62% of the patients were free of any endocrinopathy. However, this is not always the case because, despite chelation, endocrine complications may still occur in some patients [102].

## Transfusion-transmitted Infections

The risk of transfusion-transmitted infection in thalassemia patients is the same as that of other patients with multiple blood transfusions. Hepatitis C virus, HBV, HIV (human immunodeficiency virus), and syphilis are the most common sources of infection transmitted through repeated blood transfusions [4,9,99,107]. Due to the implementation of more sensitive serological methods and nucleic acid amplification tests, the residual risk of viral transmission in the EU countries and the USA significantly reduced (less than 1:1.3 million) [108]. In Africa, a high prevalence of 10% to 15% of HIV cases was related to unsafe blood transfusions [107]. Recent reports on viral infections transmitted by blood transfusion show that the rates of hepatitis C infection among Iraqis and Iranian TM patients are 23% and 19%, respectively [109,110]. Hepatitis C virus antibodies are present in 85% of multi-transfused Italian patients, 35% in the United States, 34% in France, 23% in the United Kingdom, and 21% of Indian patients [86]. Septicemia associated with contaminated blood transfusion is serious complication, such as hepatic and splenic abscesses, osteomyelitis, nephritis, meningitis, and endocarditis [89,98,100]. In the absence of specific antibiotics, the mortality rate can reach 50% of cases. Intravenous infusion of cephalosporin combined with vancomycin must be instituted. Transfusion of blood units stored for less than 2 weeks reduces the risk of microbial transfusion [93].

## Osteoporosis

The World Health Organization (WHO) defines osteoporosis as a decrease in the bone mineral density and disruption of the bone architecture (structure) leading to an increased risk of fractures. Osteopenia (a precursor to osteoporosis) and osteoporosis are important causes of morbidity in thalassemic patients in males and females. In TM, a decrease in bone mass can occur due to increased bone resorption and/or decreased bone formation, both of which may lead to osteopenia, osteoporosis, and microfractures [6,8,112,113]. These events are sequelae to hyperplasia of the erythroid bone marrow and expansion of the marrow cavity. Other factors associated with TM bone loss include delayed sexual maturity, decreased growth hormone, hypoparathyroidism, diabetes, hypothyroidism, and liver disease. Much of osteopathy is associated with inadequate transfusion and chelating therapy [111-113]. Iron depots within bones may lead to impairments in osteoblast activity and enhancement of osteoclasts activity [6,8,113]. This provides the rationale for the use of bisphosphonates, which are potent inhibitors of osteoclast function and can be used to treat TM-induced osteoporosis [114]. According to reports, the incidence of osteoporosis in TM patients is between 52% and 90%, and the incidence of bone fracture is 65% to 70% higher than that of the general population [112,115]. The incidence of osteopenia and bone fracture in TM patients was 22.6% and 16.6%, respectively [116]. Osteoporosis is related to the onset and development of periodontal disease [117].

# MANAGEMENT

At the first presentation, it is essential to obtain the social and medical history of the affected family to assess the pattern of inheritance and to provide counseling on the possible course of the disease, management, and the risk of having further thalassemic children. Management of patients with TM lay under the following headings: (1) Life-long blood transfusion to correct anemia and suppress erythropoiesis. (2) Chelation therapy balances the rate of iron accumulations resulted from a blood transfusion and inhibition of gastrointestinal iron absorption by increasing iron excretion. (3) Splenectomy may be necessary because an overactive spleen(hypersplenism) increases the need for blood transfusion and inhibit chelation therapy to control iron levels. (4) Management of iron overload that causes endocrinopathies, cardiac disease, and osteoporosis. (5) Control the infection caused by hypersplenism or splenectomy. (6) Bone marrow transplantation (BMT). Gene therapy offers a potential cure for β-thalassemia and would represent an ideal alternative to both conventional therapy and BMT [102,118-120]. The survival rate of TM has been significantly improved followed by the judicious use of blood transfusion and effective chelation therapy to control the iron accumulation caused by blood transfusion and associated with severe and lethal effects.

## Splenectomy

The main function of the spleen is to filter blood. It has a variety of auxiliary functions in the body, including removing microorganisms and antigens from the bloodstream, removing old or damaged blood cells, producing antibodies (mainly immunoglobulin M), and conducting immune responses by detecting pathogens. The excessive function of the spleen in TM can cause splenomegaly, which worsens anemia by reducing the lifespan of the transfused RBCs and intensifies the need for blood transfusions, thus exacerbating the problems caused by iron accumulations. Many TM patients who rely on blood transfusions require splenectomy. The main therapeutic principles of splenectomy are: (1) Prevent the development of extramedullary hematopoiesis (production of blood cells) by increasing hemoglobin levels. (2) Prolong RBCs survival by reducing the number of RBCs removed from circulation. (3) Reduces the need for blood transfusions. (4) Decrease iron overload [9,100-102]. Splenectomy is recommended when: (1). The annual transfusion requirement is greater than 200–220 mL RBC/kg of body weight per year with a hematocrit of 70%. The normal hematocrit levels of children aged 6 to 12 years are 35% to 45%. (2). The annual blood need exceeds 1.5 times those of splenectomized patients [89,102]. Because of the risk of post-splenectomy infection, splenectomy should delay until the age of 5 years or later [93,97]. Taher *et al.* [97] suggested that splenectomy may reduce the body's ability to scavenge toxic free iron species. The indications for splenectomy among patients with β-thalassemia are becoming increasingly restrictive.

## Endocrinopathies

Endocrine dysfunction is a common and serious complication of TM, which requires prompt recognition and treatment.  Delayed growth and pubertal development, abnormal gonadal functions, impaired thyroid, parathyroid and adrenal functions, diabetes, and disorderly bone growth are commonly encountered. Early detection and adoption of appropriate blood transfusion regimens, chelation therapy, and treatment of complications are the keys to management. Due to TM hypogonadism (40% to 80% of males), patients suffer from growth retardation, puberty failure, sexual dysfunction, and infertility [3-5,86]. These problems are caused by chronic anemia, excessive iron deposition in the pituitary gland and testes. Iron deposition on gonadotroph cells of the pituitary leads to disruption of gonadotropin, LH (luteinizing hormone), and FSH (follicle-stimulating hormone) production [3,89,106]. Delayed pubertal growth and sexual development may occur despite the timely initiation of iron chelation in early childhood. If pubertal changes have not developed by 13 years of age in females or 16 years of age in males, the use of gonadotropin-releasing hormone and gonadal steroids has been suggested [102]. Because hormonal treatment of pubertal disorders in thalassemia may associate with complications, each patient has to be assessed individually.

## Blood Transfusion

Blood transfusion therapy is the main treatment for patients with severe β-thalassemia, usually starting around 2 years of age. Goals include correcting anemia, inhibiting bone marrow activity to produce ineffective erythropoiesis, delaying the development of splenomegaly, inhibiting the intestinal absorption of iron, promoting normal growth, and allowing normal physical activity [2,9,10,89]. In addition, regular blood transfusions can treat the hypoxic symptoms of anemia and maintain Hb levels at 13-14 g/dL after transfusion. Hb after blood transfusion prevents growth disorders, organ damage, skeletal deformities, and allows normal activity and quality of life [89,111,107]. However, Hb greater than 14-15 g/dL after blood transfusion has the risk of high viscosity and stroke. Before the first transfusion, patients' RBCs are typed for Rh and ABO antigens. Parents and first-degree relatives should not be blood donors for these candidates. Hepatitis B vaccination should be given before transfusion therapy [102]. Currently, there is no vaccine against hepatitis C.

To start a blood transfusion, patients with TM should have severe anemia (Hb<7 g/dL) for more then two weeks. In addition, other factors associated with TM anemia and should be considered are facial changes, poor growth, large extramedullary hematopoietic function, bone expansion, and splenomegaly [3,5,9,107]. The frequency of blood transfusion is usually once every two to four weeks. Generally, the RBCs to be infused should not exceed 15 to 20 mL/kg body weight/day and infused at a maximum rate of 5 mL/kg/hour to avoid a rapid increase in blood volume. A moderate transfusion regimen may reduce iron loading in TM without producing an excessive expansion of erythropoiesis [120,121]. While regular transfusions greatly contribute to the quality and length of life of TM patients, they also leave the body with an iron overload.

## Iron Chelation

Iron chelating therapy should be provided to all TM patients who require long-term blood transfusions to reduce iron load and prevent and/or delay complications related to iron deposition in the tissues. Iron chelation therapy doubles the life expectancy of transfusion-dependent TM patients [5,7,9,121]. This therapy balances the rate of iron accumulation in the blood transfusion by increasing iron excretion in the urine and faces. Patients who are pregnant or breastfeeding should avoid chelating agents. Ideally, chelating therapy should be started before clinically iron accumulates. Patients who have received multiple blood transfusions without adequate chelation can also be treated, but they may require an intensive chelation regimen [118]. Since chelating agents remove iron from the heart much slower than iron from the liver, prolonged intensive iron chelation therapy is usually required. The dose of an iron-chelating agent is determined by the presence or absence of cardiac iron overload, the rate of transfusional iron loading, and the body iron burden. The greater the rate of transfusional iron loading, the greater the dose of an iron chelator is needed to control the accumulation of iron. Patients whose iron load exceeds 7 to 15 mg iron per gram of liver are at increased risk of liver fibrosis, diabetes mellitus, and other complications, and require more intensive iron-chelation therapy.

Administration of a chelator usually starts at the age of 2-4 years that requires an infusion of 20- 25 RBC units, and the serum ferritin level is greater than 1000 µg/dL [3,5,9,24]. There are 3 types of iron-chelating agents, namely deferoxamine (Desferal®) parenteral administration and 2-orally administered chelators;

deferiprone (L1®) and deferasirox (Exjade®) [122-124]. The key points of ideal iron chelation therapy include slow metabolism, ability to penetrate tissues and cells and chelate toxic iron species, non-toxic, affordable, availability for oral administration, and high chelation efficiency. Compliance with iron chelation therapy is necessary to control complications related to iron overload. The effectiveness of chelation is related to the dose prescribed, adherence to treatment, blood transfusion rate, variability in absorption, metabolism of the drug, or a combination of these and other factors.

## Deferoxamine (DFO)

Iron chelation therapy began in the 1960s, and DFO was the first drug used to treat iron overload in patients with TM. It is a hexadentate iron chelator, in which 1 molecule of DFO binds 1 molecule of iron, making it metabolically inactive [3,9,118]. About 100 mg of DFO binds 8 mg iron.  Having a short plasma half-life of 20–30 minutes, DFO should be administered over a span of 8-10 hours a day, on 5-7 days a week. Oral ascorbic acid is usually prescribed at 2–3 mg/kg/day at the beginning of the infusion. DFO and is administered by continuous subcutaneous infusion with the use of a battery-operated portable pump. The dose of deferoxamine is adjusted according to the body's iron load and age, ranging from 20 to 50 mg/kg body weight /day. Iron is excreted in feces (40%) and urine (60%) with 30 to 70 mg of iron is removed every day [10,121,124]. DFO treatment is inconvenient, time-consuming, and not suitable for children under 3 years of age because of its potential toxicity that may affect bones and growth. The most frequent adverse effects of DFO are local reactions at the site of infusion, skeletal changes, ocular and auditory disturbances, sometimes fever, chills, and malaise.

## Deferiprone (DFP)

This is the second-generation iron chelator launched in 1999. It obtained a full license in Europe in 2002 and was approved as a second-line drug for patients who cannot tolerate DFO infusions proved to be ineffective or have toxic reactions. It is suitable for children ≥ 6 years of age and can replace DFO when cardiac function is improved [102,122]. DFP is a bidentate chelating agent, in which 3 molecules of DFP are bound to1 molecule of iron. It has a short half-life of 3 to 4 hours, and it must be taken 3 times a day. The dose of DFP is 75-100 mg/kg body weight/day, taken orally in 3 divided doses with meals. Bounded iron is mainly excreted through urine. DFP penetrates cell membranes more rapidly than DFO. Patient compliance is excellent compared with DFO and is much less expensive than an infusion pump. Comparative studies have shown that, at comparable doses, DFP may be as effective as DFO in removing iron from the body, and is superior to DFO in reducing cardiac iron levels [121-125]. Generally, hexadentate chelators form the most stable iron chelates, while bidentate chelator agents form the least stable. Adverse effects of DFP include arthralgia, nausea, vomiting, and other gastrointestinal symptoms. The most serious adverse reactions associated with DFP are agranulocytosis and neutropenia [3,10,89].

## Deferasirox (DFX)

DFX is the latest iron-chelating drug licensed in 2006 and is available in the form of dispersed tablets.DFX is tridentate that binds iron in a 2:1 ratio [10,123,124], *i.e.*, 2 molecules of DFX bind to one molecule of iron. It has a longer half-life (8 to 16 hours) than other chelating agents. Due to its relatively long half-life, it can be administered once a day. The initial dosage is 20 mg/kg/day, which can be increased to 40 mg/kg/day based on the serum ferritin levels. Iron is excreted through feces. In the United States, this is the first-line treatment for TM patients under 2 years of age, while in Europe, DFX is approved as the first-line treatment for patients under 6 years of age. The advantages of DFX are oral administration, longer half-life (allowing for once-a-day administration), and fewer side effects [121-124].  After dissolving in water, apple, or orange juice, DFX should be taken on an empty stomach to ensure sufficient bioavailability. However, compared with the other iron chelators, DFX is more expensive. Common mild side effects include transient skin rashes and gastrointestinal upset. Hepatic and renal toxicity may occur at higher doses [123-125].

## Combined Chelation Therapy

Although three iron-chelating agents can be used, some patients still fail to respond adequately to certain chelation therapies for various reasons. The adverse drug effects may prevent optimal dosing, poor adherence to treatment, and inadequate body response. Combination therapy, including the use of two chelating agents on the same day to increases the efficiency of chelation, especially in the presence of high levels of heart or liver iron [124-127]. Clinical studies have shown that it is effective to combine low-molecular-weight chelating agents that can effectively penetrate cells and high-molecular-weight chelating agents that can form a stable association with iron. The combined treatment of DFP and DFX in TM patients can be used to reduce the heart and liver iron load. Simultaneous administration of DFO and DFX can rapidly reduce systemic and myocardial iron and provide excellent control of toxic unstable plasma iron without increasing toxicity [125,126]. The combined treatment of DFO and DFP can be used to treat iron overload in patients who are sub-optimally chelated by the maximum dose of DFP. Their synergistic effect on iron balance and iron excretion can be explained by a shuttle mechanism, where DFP enters cells and removes iron, and then iron transport to DFO for excretion in urine/feces [124,126,127]. Evidence from 18 trials shows that the adverse effects increased in patients treated with DFP compared with DFO, and in patients treated with combined DFP and DFO compared with DFO alone [128].

## Osteoporosis

Osteoporosis is a progressive skeletal disorder commonly found in TM patients and is an important cause of morbidity and mortality. It is characterized by low bone mass and deterioration of the structure of bone tissue leading to an increase in bone fragility and risk of fracture. The early identification of osteoporosis is of paramount importance. Delayed diagnosis and inadequate treatment can lead to severe osteoporosis, skeletal abnormalities, fractures, spinal deformities, nerve compression, and growth failure. There is no cure for osteoporosis. Treatment aims to slow or stop bone loss and improve bone density. Effective iron chelation, proper hormone replacement (sex steroids, growth hormone), bisphosphonates therapy, improvement of Hb levels, calcium (1–1.2 gram/day), vitamin D (800 unit/day), zinc (8–11 mg/day) administration and physical activity are management of the disease. Bisphosphonates are pyrophosphate-like drugs developed in the 1980s for the treatment of bone and calcium metabolism diseases. They are the main treatment for osteoporosis because of their potent inhibitors of osteoclast-mediated bone resorption and increase bone mineral density that prevents fractures. Oral bioavailability is <1% and must be administered on an empty stomach to maximize absorption or by intravenous infusion. Oral bisphosphonates can cause mild gastrointestinal discomfort, while intravenous bisphosphonates can cause a transient fever, bone and muscle pain, and osteonecrosis of the jaw after dental surgery (such as tooth extraction).

## BMT and Genetic Treatment

Allogeneic bone marrow transplantation (BMT)or stem cell transplantation from HLA-matched related donors (HLA: human leukocyte antigen) was the first curative method reported in 1982 and is still the only definitive treatment available for patients with transfusion-dependent β-thalassemia. Since then, more than 3,000 successful transplants have been reported [102]. The purpose of this therapy is to correct ineffective erythropoiesis and hemolytic anemia, thereby eliminating the need for blood transfusions. BMT relies on high-dose chemotherapy to remove the thalassemia-producing cells in the bone marrow and replace them with healthy donor cells. Reports show that according to the stage of the disease, the incidence of the free disease is as high as 80-97% [89,102,103]. The major limitation of BMT is finding histocompatibility donors. About 25–30% of thalassemia patients could have a matched sibling donor. Complications of BMT such as postoperative infections and thromboembolic events may arise [89, 102, 129].

The gene therapy of autologous transplantation of genetically modified hematopoietic stem cells provides a new therapeutic prospect for the treatment of β-thalassemia. The goal of the therapy is to achieve a stable introduction of functional globin genes into the patient's own hematopoietic stem cells in order to correct ineffective erythropoiesis and hemolytic anemia, thus obviating the need for transfusion. This method also focuses on correcting the DNA sequence for specific mutations in the globulin gene to restore the synthesis of the globulin chain [89,118-120,129]. These methods may provide patients with a wide range of treatment options, thereby freeing patients from the traditional management of the disease, related complications, and the burden of the healthcare system. The future treatment of beta-thalassemia will depend on the benefits, risks, costs of routine blood transfusion, and iron chelation ratio. The challenge for the future is to ensure that people who are born with a severe form of thalassemia will continue to thrive. Effective screening and prevention programs eventually decrease the number of severely affected patients worldwide.

## Diet and Nutrition

### ■ Diet

There is no evidence that a low-iron diet being necessary for transfused patients on chelation therapy. The amount of iron obtained from one unit of packed red cells (200 mg) far outweighs the amount of iron obtained from the diet. Only foods rich in iron should be cut down or eat in moderation for TM patients. Much of iron is found in a variety of foods, including proteins, grains, fruits, and vegetables. Proteins that contain a high amount of iron are present in oysters, liver, shrimp, beef, beans, pork, peas, lentils, and peanut butter. Fruits rich in iron include strawberries, watermelon, figs, dates, and raisins. Vegetables high in iron are spinach, leafy green vegetables, sweet potatoes, broccoli, and beet greens. Foods that inhibit iron absorption are tea, coffee, chocolate, and soy products. Because osteoporosis is common in TM, patients must obtain plenty of calcium with vitamin D, through dairy products, fish, cheese, and green leafy vegetables. A diet rich in phosphorus and vitamin E content, such as eggs and vegetable oils is recommended.

# ■ Nutrition

Nutritional deficiencies are common in thalassemia. Malnutrition could be attributed to inadequate nutrient intake, intestinal malabsorption, and nutrient removal by iron-chelating drugs. Patients may have reduced intake of many key nutrients including vitamins, folate (or folic acid; a type of vitamin B), calcium, magnesium, and zinc [130-132]. A diet low in fresh fruits and vegetables is the main cause of folate deficiency. Optimal nutritional status is imperative for growth and development, immune function, and bone health. Vitamin C and D deficiency can lead to impaired osteoblast activation, reduced collagen synthesis, and increased bone resorption rates. Calcium and vitamin D are commonly prescribed supplements for thalassemia patients. Their deficiency is associated with poor bone mineralization, muscle weakness, and more importantly, affects the heart muscle [133]. Folic acid supplements of up to 1mg/day are needed for all patients with low hemoglobin levels. Vitamin C helps in the conversion of an insoluble form of tissue storage iron (hemosiderin) into ferritin, from which iron can be chelated and excreted. Multivitamin preparations containing iron should be avoided. Finally, the decline in physical activity levels due to disease complications and/or overprotection has a negative impact on bone renewal, resulting in decreased bone formation and increased absorption [3,8,132].

# DENTAL CARE

Dental treatment of TM patients requires special attention because the patient may suffer from complications of the disease, such as heart and liver dysfunction, diabetes, weakened immunity, and post-splenectomy infections. Medical history is essential to provide adequate dental treatment and avoid complications due to disease or treatment. Most patients with thalassemia can safely receive routine dental treatment. However, for patients with a severe form of the disease, long-term surgery should be avoided. Prior to conduct an intensive dental procedure, a thorough medical history, and current medical status are required for general health assessment. This should include •Hb level. •chelating agents and other drugs such as antibiotics. •history of splenectomy. •patient prognosis. •life expectancy. Complex surgical treatment is contraindicated if blood transfusion and chelation therapy are not under control. Close contact with the hematology team must determine possible complications during extensive dental treatment and the necessary measures to determine safe outcomes. Treatment should never be initiated during a crisis unless in an emergency situation, and treatment should be designed to decrease infection and discomfort. Dental and medical practitioners and health care professionals, especially those working in multi-ethnic communities, need to understand the nature and source of this disease and its impact on general and oral health.

Patients who undergo splenectomy are susceptible to sepsis. To prevent bacteremia-causing dental treatment, prophylactic preoperative and postoperative antibiotics should prescribe. Any invasive dental procedures in these patients should be performed after a blood transfusion with a hemoglobin level of more than 10 g/dL. Antibiotic prophylaxis similar to that used for the prevention of bacterial endocarditis should be administered. That is, 50 mg/kg of amoxicillin (maximum dose 2 g) one hour before dental work. If the patient is sensitive to penicillin, 20 mg/kg of clindamycin (maximum dose of 600 mg) is the alternative regimen. Some of the medications to avoid are sulfa drugs, chloramphenicol, ciprofloxacin, doxycycline, and aspirin. Paracetamol is a safe alternative to aspirin. The radiographic absence of the inferior dental (alveolar) canal borders in many TM patients should be considered to avoid injury of the inferior alveolar nerve during surgical operations of the posterior mandibular teeth and implant placement. Elective surgery, such as removing asymptomatic teeth, should be avoided. Thalassemic patients are at risk of viral hepatitis due to blood transfusions from donors infected by the Hepatitis C virus. Thus, appropriate precautions should be taken by the dental team when these patients are to be treated.

## Dental Caries and Periodontal Disease

Patients with TM are at risk for dental caries and periodontal disease, associated with poor oral hygiene and dental care negligence. Other factors of the high incidence of caries and/or periodontal disease in these patients are reduced salivary flow rate, lower level of salivary immunoglobulin, high count of pathogenic bacteria (Streptococcus mutans in caries and Actinomycetemcomitans in periodontitis), mouth breathing, malocclusion, malnutrition, underlying systemic condition, infection, and impaired immune system. Therefore, patients should be kept under an intensive preventive program with regular follow-up. In some cases, a three-month recall may be necessary. Patients need proper oral hygiene instructions and motivation, including brushing their teeth and using chlorhexidine rinses or gels. For children where manual dexterity is limiting, the use of electric brushes is recommended. Effective prophylaxis, fluoride therapy, and fissure sealant should be applied to minimize the future need for extensive dental procedures. Professional fluoride therapy should be provided at 3 months' intervals and fluoride varnish is the best choice for children under the age of 6 years. Due to the impaired immune function of these patients, the risk of infection after endodontic treatment should be assessed. Primary teeth with infected pulp should be removed, do not try pulp therapy. Extractions should perform under antibiotic coverage.

## Orthodontic Treatment

Orthodontic treatment for the TM patient is strictly elective. These patients often have malocclusion or skeletal abnormalities. Correction of proclined maxillary anterior teeth and increased overjet may undertake to improve aesthetics, reduce susceptibility to trauma, avoid gingival inflammation, improve functional capacity and children's self-esteem. Orthodontic treatment should begin as early as possible concentrating on preventive and interceptive approaches. Orthodontic appliances should be appropriately designed to prevent irritation and bacterial infections of soft tissues. Due to the thin cortex and increased bone remodeling, less force should be applied. Because the teeth move faster than normal, it is necessary to closely follow up patients at short intervals between appointments. Smaller tooth size, short and spiky roots, and reduced dental arch dimensions in TM patients should be considered in planning orthodontic treatment. However, the disease may compromise the outcome of the planned treatment.

**Anesthesia and Sedation**

Most patients with TM can be treated normally using a local anesthetic as long as the dose is limited to one to two cartridges. Because of the possibility of impaired local circulation, a short procedure can be performed using an anesthetic without a vasoconstrictor. If the procedure requires long, profound anesthesia using 2% Lidocaine with vasoconstrictor epinephrine or adrenaline, 1:80,000 (0.012 mg) is preferred. If necessary, nitrous oxide/oxygen can be used. Conscious sedation is a technique in which the use of a drug or drugs produces a state of depression of the CNS, enabling treatment to be administered. Throughout the period of sedation, verbal contact with the patient is maintained.

Nitrous oxide/oxygen ($N_2O/O_2$) is widely accepted as a behavioral management technique for pediatric dentistry, usually using 30% nitrous oxide and 70% oxygen or 50/50 anesthesia intensity. It is a colorless, odorless gas of sweet smell, non-irritant, causing a feeling of euphoria. It is an effective analgesic/anti-anxiety drug that can cause depression in the central nervous system (CNS) and has little effect on the respiratory system. Nitrous oxide is quickly absorbed, and it can take effect and recover quickly within two to three minutes. It causes minimal impairment of any reflexes, thus protecting the cough reflex. Among other organizations, the American Academy of Pediatric Dentistry (AAPD), recognizes that nitrous oxide/oxygen inhalation sedation is a safe and effective technique to reduce anxiety, produce analgesia, and enhance effective communication between a patient and health care provider. Nitrous oxide is a weak general anesthetic. In general anesthesia, it is used in a 2:1 ratio with oxygen for a more powerful general anesthetic effect.

<u>Midazolam</u> (Versed®) belongs to the sedative class of benzodiazepines. Midazolam is one of the most commonly used drugs for conscious sedation in pediatric dentistry, an aid to behavior management techniques, a drug to manage seizures during dental treatment, and as premedication in general anesthesia. It is a powerful, short-acting hypnotic sedative that can cause drowsiness and reduces anxiety (anxiolytic). It also has anticonvulsant, amnestic (memory loss), and muscle relaxant properties. When taken orally, it is rapidly absorbed in the gastrointestinal tract, producing a peak effect of about 30 minutes, and has a short half-life of 1.5-2.5 hours. The half-life in children is lesser than in adults due to the fact that children have more active liver enzymes. In contrast to midazolam, the half-life of diazepam is 24 to 40 hours. Half-life refers to the time required for the plasma concentration of a drug to decrease to half of its original value. Oral midazolam in

doses between 0.5 to 0.75 mg /kg of body weight to be provided 15 to 30 minutes before treatment. Like other CNS depressants, midazolam may cause respiratory depression. After administrating midazolam, continuous monitoring of respiratory and heart function is necessary until the patient is stable. This must be done in a clinical or hospital setting. Precautions for using midazolam in patients with asthma and epilepsy. Serious and life-threatening reactions may occur in some patients, including airway obstruction, apnea, hyperventilation, and hypotension. Routes of the administration include intravenous (IV), intramuscular (IM), oral, rectal, sublingual, and nasal. It is available as a syrup (2 mg/ml) or injectable vials (1 mg/ 1 mL or 5 mg/1 mL). The recommended dose of midazolam in children differs per the route of administration. Flumazenil in a dose of 0.01 mg/kg/dose IV is an antidote, which reverses the sedative effect of Midazolam.

## General Anesthesia

In TM, not only the problems caused by the severity of anemia itself, but also problems related to blood transfusion treatment and bone deformation that may complicate tracheal intubation should be considered. Patients with TM may require elective or emergency surgery, such as therapeutic splenectomy, cholecystectomy, correction of facial deformities, fractures, and dental surgery [134]. For surgery, a comprehensive clinical examination and laboratory tests are required, including underlying pathologies, iron overload, chelation therapy, and other medications. It is very important to evaluate the airway. A difficulty may be faced in placing the mask ventilation and intubation due to maxillofacial deformities in about 2/3rd. Maxillary hypertrophy occurs in 24.9% of nasal airway problems in 16.7% of the patients (Table **1**). TM patients have smaller upper and middle pharyngeal airway spaces and short vertical pharyngeal length [135], which may be problematic when preparing for anesthesia.

Due to TM anemia and hypoxia, appropriate Hb levels must be obtained through blood transfusion before general anesthesia. This should be done 10 to 15 days before the operation. For children, optimal Hb levels obtained after a blood transfusion should be in the range of 10-12 g/dL. There is no recommendation for discontinuing iron chelation therapy before surgery. Patients with TM have a low immune function and are prone to infections, so broad-spectrum antibiotics should be used during the perioperative period. The choice of anesthetic techniques and drugs should be case-specific, according to the planned surgery and patient's condition. Both general and neuraxial anesthesia has been used safely in TM patients. Standard intravenous, inhalational agents, and opioids have been administered for induction and maintenance of anesthesia with no adverse reactions

[134]. The most common inhalation anesthetics are nitrous oxide, sevoflurane, or desflurane.

## Psychological Adjustment

Patients with thalassemia are prone to psychological challenges; including depression, anxiety, and poor quality of life, which can affect the patient's motivation and willingness to accept dental treatment. TM is a chronic disease that is considered a major health problem in the public health system due to the high cost of treatment involving regular blood transfusions, iron chelation, frequent hospitalizations, and general medical follow-up. On the other hand, this places a burden on the affected families and their children, making them more vulnerable to emotional, social, psychological, and behavioral problems. Due to the underlying chronic anemia in TM, patients may experience fatigue, dizziness, shortness of breath, headache, and leg cramps. Psychological support should be tailored to the patient's age and their toleration of the planned procedure on the day of treatment. The appointment should be made as short as possible to reduce stress.

## Bisphosphonates-related Osteonecrosis

Oral bisphosphonates are the most commonly used for the treatment of osteoporosis. As an effective osteoclast inhibitor, bisphosphonates can slow down the remodeling process, thereby increasing bone mineral density [136-138]. Remodeling is essential for bone healing, and the inhibitory effect of bisphosphonates can impair bone healing. Osteonecrosis of the jawbones is a complication of bisphosphonates (BP) therapy, which is characterized by the mucosal exposed area of the jawbone that does not heal within 6-8 weeks [137]. The risk factor for bisphosphonate-related osteonecrosis of the jaw (BRONJ) is dentoalveolar surgery; such as teeth extractions, periapical surgery, trauma, dental implants, periodontal surgery involving osseous injury, and poor oral hygiene. About two-thirds of the confirmed cases involved the mandible, and the rest involved the maxilla. Signs and symptoms include pain, infection, swelling, paraesthesia, suppuration, sinus tracts, poor healing, and non-specific radiological abnormalities (Fig. **22**). Recent studies have shown that intravenous of BP into cancer patients can cause BRONJ in 20% of patients. The prevalence of BRONJ related to oral BP account for less than 0.3% of individuals. Higher incidence in patients taking high-dose intravenous bisphosphonates. On average, patients taking oral bisphosphonates develop BRONJ after 4.6 years [136, 137].

Prior to initiating bisphosphonate therapy, patients should receive a thorough dental examination and radiographic evaluation. Teeth with a poor prognosis should be extracted, and any other dental surgical procedures should be completed before bisphosphonate therapy. For patients who have been treated with bisphosphonates, restorative and non-surgical treatments are safe. The main management includes antibacterial mouth rinses, antibiotics, superficial debridement, and discontinuation of oral bisphosphonates.

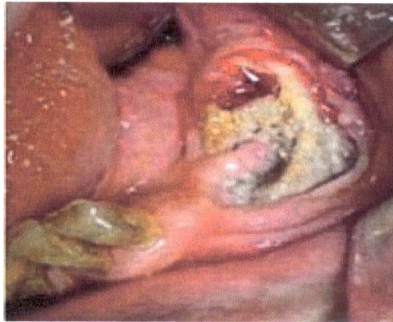

**Fig. (22)**. Clinical presentation of bisphosphonates-related osteonecrosis of the mandible showing mucosal exposure of the necrotic bone [Courtesy of Prof. Angel Bakardjiev. J Dent Oro Surg. 2016;1(4):121].

# PREVENTION PROGRAMS

Hemoglobinopathies are the most common monogenic disorders in humans, among them thalassemia constitutes a serious medical and public health problem in high prevalence regions. Hb disorders present a significant health problem in 71% of 229 countries. Over 330,000 affected infants are born annually (83% sickle cell disorders, 17% thalassemias). Hb disorders account for about 3.4% of deaths in children less than 5 years of age [12]. Screening for Hb disorders should form part of basic health services in most countries. Thalassemia is common in countries of the Mediterranean, Southeast Asia, the Middle East, the Indian subcontinent, and North Africa [12-14,139]. Patients with TM placed a burden on the healthcare systems in these countries and brought serious medical, social, and economic problems to the patients and their families. In North America and Northern European countries, the disease is traditionally rare. The flow of migration has led to an increase in the number of patients in the area. However, the COVID-19 pandemic has greatly reduced migration, but its long-term consequences remain to be seen. Although significant progress has been made in the treatment of β-thalassemia, many challenges still need to be overcome before global disease control can be achieved. Preventing the birth of new cases of thalassemia is considered the best way to control the disease. Detecting carriers of thalassemia and informing them of the risk and the possibility of reducing the risk will lead to a decrease in the number of births and deaths of children with the disease.

Implementing appropriate prevention programs, including premarital counseling, is essential for the transition from the treatment of children at risk to the prevention of childbirth. This allows individuals to receive information about their health and the potential health risks of their offspring. Prevention can be achieved through the following methods:

- Population education and awareness,
- Providing genetic counseling to the carriers and parents of children with thalassemia,
- Detection carriers through large-scale screening of high-risk communities,
- Prenatal genetic test [139,140-143].

Effective public education is the first step in any prevention program. The first attempts at large-scale and national prevention programs were adopted by Italian provinces, Greece, Cyprus, and Sardinia from the 1970s. The program is characterized by intensive education of the health personnel and the population at large, including secondary school and university students to raise their awareness of the disease. It makes use of mass media, posters, and booklets. The information includes the genetics of the disease, the nature of the disease, clinical problems, treatments, complications, and life expectancy. Premarital thalassemia screening was carried out, as part of a school prevention programme. In the above-mentioned countries/regions, educational programs, screening, and genetic counseling for at-risk groups have greatly reduced the number of newborns with TM from 1:250 to 1:4000 [139,140]. The main prevention programs established in many countries in Europe, Asia, and Australia are often drawn from the experience of Sardinia.

If public education is provided, the knowledge and understanding of screening for carriers of thalassemia can be improved. Prior to testing, individual or population should be provided with appropriate information about thalassemia to determine whether to conduct genetic screening at the same time as counseling. Carrier screening is performed after obtaining informed consent. The World Health Organization guidelines (1998), stated that no compulsory genetic testing should be carried out [144]. Several countries, mostly Mediterranean and Arab countries, such as Cyprus, Iran, Saudi Arabia, UAE, Bahrain, Jordan, Palestine, Qatar, and other countries have passed laws that require all couples to be screened for hemoglobinopathies before marriage in order to restrict the spread of the disease. Genetic tests can be applied to individuals in the context of health care, or to populations in the context of public health programs. In many countries with limited resources, screening and prevention programs are not enough, and access to effective treatment is far from universal. Carriers can be detected by Hb electrophoresis and/or high-performance liquid chromatography [3,4,23,145].

**Premarital Testing**

The premarital screening and genetic counseling program aims to reduce thalassemia births in the following ways: 1. Prevention of at-risk marriages through discouragement during counseling. 2. Reduce or prevent congenital disorders caused by the mother-to-child transmission of genetic or infectious diseases. 3. Alleviates anxiety especially if there is a family history of certain genetic diseases or marriage within relatives. 4. Through proper diagnosis and consultation, the family's financial, physical, and psychological burden can be reduced. It has been suggested that screening can reduce the burden of thalassemia by reducing risky marriages and preventing up to 95% of births [146,147]. The programs can also be divided by timing testing in relation to pregnancy being either pre-pregnancy or in the early stages of pregnancy. There are more options available to a couple if screening has occurred before conception. Couples can decide to terminate their relationship, or they can choose to continue the prenatal diagnosis during the first-trimester of pregnancy. If the fetus is affected by TM, they can choose to terminate the pregnancy [139,141-143]. Many countries do allow termination of pregnancy due to fetal abnormalities, including China, Cuba, Cyprus, India, Sri Lanka, and South Africa [148]. Iran conducts premarital screening for thalassemia and allows abortion in the first 16 weeks of pregnancy [149]. There are considerable differences in the attitude of people toward screening and for prenatal diagnosis and termination of pregnancy. Cultural, religious, ethical, and legal considerations must be considered in each country. In Muslim-majority countries, the analysis of abortion laws has proven to be a conservative approach. Among 47 countries, 18 countries legally allow abortion only in situations that threaten the life of pregnant women [150].

## Strategies for Prevention

The best way to control the disease is to prevent the birth of new cases of thalassemia. In developing countries, there is a need for in-depth education of health professionals and the public in the field of preventive genetics, development of national plans for care and prevention, and the support from health organizations and funding agencies of these initiatives [139,151]. Strategies for prevention include [152]:

• Integrate community counseling and screening programs into primary health care. This requires the education and training of primary health workers.

• Educate the public by updating high school curricula and mass media education activities about local culture and religious beliefs.

• Strengthen human resources by updating medical and nursing college courses related to the practice of human genetics, as well as guidelines on how to deal with common genetic and congenital diseases.

• Initiation of population screening programs and national birth registries.

• Introduce new technologies and strengthen existing genetic services.

## Cost of Treatment

Patients with severe β-thalassemia need life-long treatment to prevent and control the clinical consequences of the disease. The cost for the treatment includes a regular blood transfusion, chelation therapy, laboratory tests, and tests of heart, kidney, and liver function. For many people and public medical systems around the world, the cost of providing medical services to sick patients is unaffordable [7,120]. At present, about 100,000 patients receive regular transfusions for β-thalassemia worldwide. In some countries, the need for blood transfusion therapy for patients can be a huge burden. In Greece, the cost of produce one unit of blood is estimated to be 130 Euro, Iran 25 USD, and India 14.5 USD. About 33% to 47% of the treatment costs of patients with TM are due to blood transfusions. Iron chelation therapy accounts for approximately half (43–55%) of the total current cost of treatment [120]. In resource-poor countries, only 12% of children with transfusion-dependent thalassemia received appropriate blood transfusion therapy, while <40% of transfusion patients received appropriate iron chelation therapy.

## ■ Developed Countries

In the United Kingdom, the total healthcare cost of managing TM in the past 50 years is estimated at 483,454 pounds (USD720,200). If half of the patients receives bone marrow transplantation, the cost can be reduced by as much as 37% [153]. Lifetime treatment costs for 600 registered TM patients in the UK range from 188,000 to 226,000 pounds [154]. The US report (2017) shows that the average annual blood transfusion cost per patient/year is USD 22,478, and the cost of chelation therapy is USD 52,718 [155]. Cost-utility analysis in the UK indicated that deferiprone is the most cost-effective chelator for iron overload in patients with TM [156]. In Canada, the total cost of Deferasirox during the lifetime of patients with β-thalassemia is USD 571,156, while the cost of Deferoxamine is USD 445,139 [157]. The iron chelation therapy accounts for about half of the total current cost of treatment for patients with TM.

## ■ Developing Countries

The cost of treating thalassemia in some developing countries has been reviewed [158]. In India, depending on age and the presence of complications, the cost of supportive care and management for TM children ranges from USD 629 to USD 2300 per year, with an average of USD 1135. Nearly half this amount is used for drug therapy [15]. In Iran, the cost of care for 46 TM patients approximately USD 300,000 annually, and 3 million USD for a ten-year program. Caring for 235 cases could reach up to USD 15,275,000 in 10 years [159]. In Thailand, the lifetime cost of treating β-thalassemia children is around USD 149,900 over a period of 30 years. The cost-benefit ratio of screening and treatment was found to be 72:1 [158].

## Cost-benefits of preventive programs

The burden of screening procedures and the use of molecular analysis to detect carriers as well as treating β-thalassemia patients are heavy as compared to the low prevention cost. Population education and awareness, the use of posters and brochures, and the training of health personnel are key factors for the success of prevention programs. Analysis carried out in Israel showed that the cost of preventing an affected newborn with β-thalassemia was USD 63, 660, while the cost of treating a patient during the life expectancy of 50 years is USD 1,971,380 (average annual cost: USD 39,427). Thus, the prevention of 45 affected newborns over a ten-year period is a net saving of USD 88.5 million to the health budget [160, 161]. A number of studies have shown that the cost of screening and prenatal diagnostic procedures is much lower than the cost of treatment for patients with thalassemia [12, 120, 161, 162].

## SUMMARY AND RECOMMENDATIONS

Thalassemia syndrome is a group of inherited hemolytic anemia disorders that involve defects in Hb production. Severeβ-thalassemia (TM) is inherited *via* two mutated genes, one from each parent. It presents in childhood, usually between the ages of six months and one year. Children who do not receive TM treatment will die in their first decade, while those who receive irregular blood transfusions will usually die before the second or third decade. The main treatment for TM is regular blood transfusion at intervals of 2–4 week. This will treat anemia, suppress ineffective erythropoiesis (RBCs formation), enable children to develop, and prolong survival. Coupled with blood transfusions and iron overload, iron chelation is essential in the treatment of TM. Life-long care is needed, and financial support should be provided for appropriate treatment. Nowadays, autologous transplantation of genetically modified hematopoietic stem cells represents a novel therapeutic promise.

Based on current data, the following conclusions and recommendations can be drawn:

1. Patients with TM are at high risk for dental caries and susceptible to periodontal disease. Effective preventive measures should be taken to reduce the need for extensive dental procedures. These include periodic prophylaxis, fluoride application, fissure sealant, and oral hygiene instructions.

2. Reduction in tooth crown size and dental arches in TM patients has an impact on the occlusal relationships. The patient's tooth development and growth patterns are significantly delayed. These changes should be considered in planning orthodontic treatment and orthognathic surgery.

3. In the surgical operation of the mandibular posterior teeth, the lack of imaging of the inferior alveolar canal borders in many TM patients should be considered. Precautions must be taken to avoid damage to the inferior dental nerve.

4. TM patients with acute dental infections/abscesses should receive urgent dental care and antibiotic coverage, especially if they have had a splenectomy.

5. Patients who have had a splenectomy are at high risk of massive infect-ion and bacteremia. Before the invasive procedure, antibiotic prophylaxis used for the prevention of bacterial endocarditis should be instituted.

6. Dental treatment of patients with thalassemia requires special attention, because the patient may suffer from complications of the disease; such as heart and liver dysfunction, infection, diabetes, decreased immunity, and infection. Prior to intensive dental treatment, close contact with the hematology team is required to determine potential complications.

7. The complications of TM increase with age. Early diagnosis and management allow a more favorable prognosis.

8. Successful management depends on regular blood transfusion, iron chelation, infection control, and therapeutic facilities. Compliance with chelation therapy is a key factor in the treatment of iron overload.

9. Children and adults with thalassemia should receive all recommended vaccinations, including influenza, pneumococcal, and meningococcal vaccines.

10. The cost of screening and prenatal diagnostic procedures is much lower than the cost of treating patients with thalassemia. Effective prevention strategies should be implemented in Arab countries.

11. Unless the marriage of thalassemia carriers (especially between relatives) isceased, public education and awareness of genetic diseases are strengthened, and premarital screening, genetic counseling, and prenatal diagnosis are provided, the prevention of thalassemia cannot be achieved.

# ARABIAN GULF AND NEIGHBORING COUNTRIES

In the Gulf region, hereditary hemoglobinopathies, especially thalassemia and sickle cell disease, are common, causing great suffering to sick children and an economic burden on the healthcare system. This involves two main factors: (1) The consanguineous marriage, which is associated with a high prevalence of recessively inherited disorders. (2) Marriages at a young age and large family sizes, which increase the number of affected children. Obstacles to prevention and care initiatives include insufficient genetic knowledge in the health sector and a lack of public awareness of genetic risks and the possibility of preventing these disorders. These factors, combined with certain cultural, legal, and religious restrictions, limit the selective abortion of affected fetuses [142,151,152].

## Iraq

In Iraq, there are 19 hereditary blood diseases centers, with a total of 13,500 patients. Services are provided free of charge, including regular blood transfusion and iron-chelating therapy. National guidelines for the management and prevention of hemoglobinopathies have been developed. The carrier rate of β-thalassemia in various regions of the country is between 3.7% and 4.5% [14,163,164]. In 2008, a five-year premarital screening, genetic counseling, and prenatal diagnosis (PND) program was implemented to identify carriers of hemoglobinopathies in the Kurdistan region of northern Iraq [163,165,166]. Screening is mandatory by law. A total of 102,554 individuals (51,277 couples) visiting a premarital center in Dohuk province between 2008 and 2012 were screened for carrier status and counselling. The main problems facing the program are the low public awareness of genetic diseases, the high rate of marriage among close relatives, the high cost of PND, and the short time between mandatory testing and actual marriage. In addition, some couples are not convinced by the results of the screening tests provided to them. Data on 198 high-risk couples showed that 90% of them continued their marriage plan, while 15% of married couples decided to receive PND in subsequent pregnancies. The premarital program managed to reduce the affected birth rate by 21% [165].

In Sulaimaniyah Province, a total of 108,264 people (54,132 couples) were screened for hemoglobinopathies. A follow-up survey was conducted on 130 couples suffering from β-thalassemia, and the results showed that almost all (98%) who were diagnosed through premarital screening chose to continue their marriage after counseling. The majority (76%) who underwent PND and had an affected fetus choose to terminate the pregnancy. According to reports, the number of affected births has been reduced by 65% during the five years of the implementation of the plan [166]. Despite premarital counseling provided, the number of couples who decided to continue with their marriage arrangements is quite similar to that reported in Saudi Arabia (90%) and in India (99%) [166,167].

## Saudi Arabia

In Saudi Arabia, a royal decree was passed in 2003 requiring mandatory premarital screening tests, but the decision to marry depends on the couple[10]. A study was conducted as a part of the National Premarital Screening and Genetic Counseling Program, which covered all the individuals who applied for a marriage license during the years 2004 and 2005. Of the total 488,315 individuals screened, 4.2% had a sickle cell trait, and 3.2% had a thalassemia trait [167]. Between 2004 and 2009, blood samples were obtained from the couple for genetic counseling. Among the 1,572,140 men and women examined, 4.5% were positive for sickle cell disease (carriers or cases) and 1.8% were positive for β-thalassemia. At the end of the program, the frequency of at-risk couples was reduced by about 60%, while the frequency of voluntary cancellation of marriage proposals increased by more than 5 times [168]. Between 2011 and 2015, a study was conducted on 12,30,582 people seeking marriage certificates. The results showed that the prevalence of β-thalassemia per 1,000 people was 13.6 (12.9 traits and 0.7 TM) and the incidence decreased from 24.2% in 2011 to 12% in 2015% [169]. Findings suggest that the program's objective of decreasing high-risk marriages needs further improvement of health education for the public, more efforts in counseling high-risk couples, and changes in the strategy of screening timing in regard to marriage plans [167,168].

## United Arab Emirates

In the United Arab Emirates (UAE), a decree was issued by Sheikh Hamdan Bin Rashid AI-Maktoum (1994), for establishing a thalassemia center. The health authority launched a nationwide campaign to promote premarital screening under the slogan "Emirate free of thalassemia" by 2012. Premarital screening is mandatory, but the final decision depends on the couples. After consultation, about half of the carrier couples chose to get married, while others decided to separate. Compared with the time before the prevention program was adopted, the number of affected births was reduced by half [17]. Termination of pregnancy with thalassemia is not practiced as a solution for the prevention of thalassemia in the UAE. In an interview of 100 couples about their attitudes toward genetic counseling, Al-Gazali [170] reported that almost half preferred consanguineous marriages and only 10% agreed with prenatal diagnosis and abortion, while 75% agreed with carrier screening and preconception diagnosis in affected families.

A retrospective study conducted in Ras Al Khaimah showed of the 17,826 individuals screened, 4.0% were positive for hemoglobinopathies and 1.05% had β-thalassemia [171]. Baysal [172] studied the DNA of 472 newborns related to UAE mothers and other age groups. He found that the frequency of β-thalassemia gene in the nationals was 8.3%, one of the highest in the Gulf region, and the gene mutations are more than in countries of the Mediterranean, Europe, Southeast Asia, South America, and North Africa [172]. In conclusion, Al-Gazali (2005) stated that "Effective genetic counseling in this community requires an informed educated population and introduction of carrier screening and preconception diagnosis in affected families" [170].

## Oman

According to the Ministry of Health, 75% of patients visiting the healthcare centers suffer from blood-inherited disorders. A survey conducted on 6342 children under 5 years of age, showed that the prevalence of sickle cell trait was 5.8%, and the prevalence of severe β-thalassemia was 2.2% [173]. Another study showed that in the population of 1.5 million in 1995, there were 1757 cases of sickle cell anemia and 243 cases of β-thalassemia major [174]. Umbilical cord blood samples of 7,837 newborns were analyzed for complete blood counts, Hb profile, and liquid chromatography. Results showed that β-globin abnormalities accounted for 9.5% of the samples with 4.8% sickle cell trait, and 2.6% β-thalassemia trait [175].

## Bahrain

In 2004, the King of Bahrain announced a law that made pre-marital counseling mandatory. It was also declared that after receiving counselling sessions, the marriage and reproduction choices are left for the couple to decide. A Ten-year study was conducted on 60,000 students in the 11th grade from 1999 to 2008. The blood samples were collected and Hb electrophoresis and high-performance liquid chromatography (HPLC) were used to measure and identify the different types of Hb abnormalities.The average prevalence rates of β-thalassemia trait and TM are 3.5% and 0.032%, respectively, which is slightly lower than those of other Gulf countries [176]. A retrospective study of 1,378 records of 9-month-old infants showed that the most common type of hemoglobinopathy was alpha-thalassemia (18.5%), followed by sickle cell trait 11.6% [177].

# Kuwait

Kuwait is located in the northeast corner of the Arabian Peninsula with a current population of 4,310,200, composed of 30% nationals and 70% expatriates. A retrospective study was conducted on 129 infants with TM in Sabah Hospital in Kuwait from 1965 to 1995. The age ranged from 2 to 84 months, with a median of 9 months. About 80% of patients are the result of first- or second cousin's marriage [178]. Analysis of 2,386 samples using Hb electrophoresis showed that the most common hemoglobinopathies were β-thalassemia minor (14%), sickle cell trait (6%), sickle cell anemia (0.9%), and β-thalassemia intermedia/major (0.8%) [179]. The frequency of the alpha thalassemia trait is approximately 40% in the Kuwaiti population [180].

# Jordan

Like the Gulf countries, hemoglobinopathies and genetic diseases in Jordan constitute a serious health problems and a major cause of disability and death. The economic burden of hemoglobinopathies is high. In Jordan, the annual cost of treatment is estimated to be about US$ 10 million [WHO-EM/NCD/068/E/12.11/134]. The traditional high consanguinity rate (50%) and large family size lead to an increase in the incidence of autosomal recessive disorders. Hamamy *et al.*, (2007) reported that the first-cousin marriages among Jordanian declined from 28.5% for marriages contracted between 1950 and 1979 to 19.5% for marriages contracted after 1980. The total fertility rate dropped from 7.4 in 1976 to 3.7 and 4.2 for urban and rural areas, respectively in 2004 [181]. In 1996, the prevalence of β-thalassemia in Northern Jordan was 5.9% [182]. Carrier frequencies of β-thalassemia, α-thalassemia, and sickle cell anemia in Jordan account for 3–6, 1–2, and 1–4%, respectively [181]. In 1998, approximately 1,000 TM patients were registered and it is expected that about about 80 new cases will be every year [24]. In June 2004, the mandatory national premarital screening for β-thalassemia carriers was officially launched [14]. The basic goals of the program include primary prevention. If both couples are diagnosed as carriers, they will get genetic counseling to explain their risk of having a sick child. As in other Arabic countries, if a positive result is found, the decision to get married or not is optional.

# Yemen

There are no national guidelines for the prevention and management of hemoglobinopathies or newborn screening programs. This is due to a lack of funding and staff. Blood samples were collected from 699 patients attending outpatient clinics in Sana'a City. Complete blood count, hemoglobin (Hb) electrophoresis, quantitation of Hb, and serum ferritin were determined.β-thalassemia is present in 31 patients (4.43%), and α-thalassemia trait in 60 patients (8.6%) [183].

## Iran

Among the eastern Mediterranean region, Iran is one of the major centers for the prevalence of β-thalassemia. It is estimated that there are between two and three million ofβ-thalassemia carriers[184]. Approximately 26,000 TM cases have been officially recorded, and the total prevalence of the disease is estimated to be 25/100,000; which makes Iran one of the most affected countries in the region [185]. Alpha thalassemia is not as prevalent as β-thalassemia. More than 47 different β-globin gene mutations are responsible for β-thalassemia [184]. The Thalassemia Prevention Program was launched in 1995 and includes premarital screening and genetic counseling programs for at-risk couples. By the end of 2001, over 2.7 million potential couples had been screened, and 10,298 of them were at risk [149]. The mean coverage rate of program was 74%. After counselling, cancellation of marriages was 53% [186], and the rest half proceed to marriage [149]. This program reduced the number of newborn cases in 2009 by 82% [186]. More than two-thirds (69%) of β-thalassemia carriers had insufficient knowledge regarding the prevention of the disease and its possible impact on their offspring. In a retrospective study that included 911 patients with β-thalassemia in Shiraz province, the 20-, 40-, and 60-year survival rates are 85%, 63%, and 54%, respectively [187]. A comparative study of 133 TM patients in Hamadan province showed that their 10-, 20- and 30-year survival rates were 98.3%, 88.4%, and 80.5%, respectively [188]. Socio-demographic and blood-related factors are significantly associated with the survival rate.

# GENETIC DISORDERS AMONG ARAB POPULATIONS

The Arab countries in the world are also known as the Arab world, or Arab nations and are comprised of 22 countries that are part of the Arab League and located in Africa and Asia. These nations have a total area of over 5 million square miles (12.9 million square kilometers). The total population of all countries is 423 million. Among these countries, Egypt is the most populous country with a population of more than 90 million. In the area, Algeria is the largest Arab country with a total area of 2,381,750 square kilometers. Bahrain has the smallest area , with an area of only 758 square kilometers. The majority of the citizens of Arab countries follow the religion of Islam. About one-quarter of the world's Muslims are Arabs. Throughout the nations, the adult literacy is under 77%, and the female literacy rates are much lower than that of men[https://worldpopulationreview. com/country-rankings/arab-countries].

The available evidence shows that congenital and genetic diseases are more common in Arab countries than in developed countries and account for a large proportion of infant mortality, morbidity, and disability in these countries [20,189-191]. The Arab population is characterized by large family size, high maternal and paternal age, and a high level of inbreeding with consanguinity rates in the range of 25-60% [19-21]. Certain disorders are common in the Arab world, including haemoglobinopathies, glucose-6-phosphate dehydrogenase deficiency. Different congenital malformations are caused by recessive genes and several inborn metabolic disorders. The increase in the incidence of hereditary diseases is mainly due to higher rates of inherited blood disorders and other autosomal recessive diseases. Among Arabs, the carrier rate of β-thalassemia is 2–15%, α-thalassemia is 2–50%, and sickle cell disease is 0.3–30% [20,190,191]. Arab populations have their "own" genetic disorders, both universal and particular and many of the genetic disorders in Arabs are confined to a country or region [191]. Nearly, one-third of the genetic disorders in Arabs result from congenital malformations and chromosomal abnormalities, which are also responsible for a significant proportion of perinatal and neonatal deaths. High fertility rates together with increased consanguineous marriages in Arab tend to increase the incidence of genetic and congenital abnormalities [20,148,152]. Of the six World Health Organization (WHO) Regions, the highest rate of severe congenital disorders and genetic diseases is found in the Eastern Mediterranean region, with affected children over 65 per 1,000 live births as opposed to 52/1,000 in Europe, North America, and Australia [193]. Of the 5.2 million births in the European Union (EU) each year, approximately 104,000 (2.5%) will be born with congenital anomalies. Down syndrome accounts for about 8 % of all congenital anomalies.

The first known category of genetic conditions is caused by chromosomal abnormalities. Almost one-third of Arab genetic diseases are caused by chromosomal abnormalities. The most common example is trisomy (triplicate)of chromosome 21 (Down syndrome, DS). According to the WHO, the estimated incidence of DS is between 1 in 1,000 to 1 in 1,100 live births worldwide. In western countries, the incidence of DS is 1.2–1.7 per 1000. A higher incidence rate of DS has been reported in Arab Gulf countries ranged from 1:319 in Dubai to 1:581 in Kuwait [Center for Arab Genomic Studies/Dubai –2013]. Besides the above-mentioned Arab family structure, factors that contribute to DS incidence in this region are the relatively high proportion of births to older mothers, and partial or complete lack of prenatal detection, which can aid parental decisions to terminate pregnancies with DS fetuses. Up to 50% of children with Down's syndrome are born to mothers aged 40 or over. In the US, 67% of pregnancies with DS are terminating. The second category of genetic diseases is caused by major mutations or highly penetrant mutations, called monogenic diseases (single-gene diseases or Mendelian diseases). There are about1,500 single-gene diseases in which genetic defects have been identified [191-194]. A review of the molecular basis of β-thalassemia in various Arab countries revealed that there are 52 mutations, most of which are from the Mediterranean and Asia. The factors that contribute to the etiology of congenital malformation include single-gene disorders, chromosome abnormalities, multifactorial inheritance, and environmental factors [192,195-197].

Monogenic disorders are classified into three main categories: dominant, recessive, and sex (X) linked. They have severe clinical manifestations, high morbidity, and early death. Approximately 30% of children with congenital or genetic diseases may die in infancy, and a similar number of children will have chronic severe disabilities. Autosomal recessive disorders are responsible for a great deal of infant mortality, morbidity, physical and mental handicaps in Arab countries [194-197]. Teebi and Farag  (1997), described genetically transmitted diseases among Arabs as follows autosomal recessive inheritance (61%), autosomal dominant (28%), and X-linked traits (6%) [194]. Later, Teebi (2010) [191] compiled a list of syndromes in the Arab population containing 160 syndromes compared with 113 syndromes in 1997. The inheritance of these syndromes is 133 (83%) autosomal recessive, 27 (17%) autosomal dominant, and 5 (3%) X-linked.

Consanguinity itself does not cause genetic disease; it only increases the chance that reproduction will occur between two carriers for the same recessive genetic diseases. Al-Gazali *et al.* (1997) found that children of consanguineous parents are more likely to enter into consanguineous marriages than children of non-consanguineous parents [196]. Hamamy *et al.* (2007) stated that the offspring of first-cousin parents were significantly more prone to marry their relatives than the offspring of non-consanguineous parents, with rates of 25.3% and 17.1%, respectively [181]. Empirical studies have shown that the incidence of morbidity in first cousin offspring is 7.5% higher than that of offspring from unrelated couples [193]. Birth defects in developing countries are >70/1000 live births, while in Europe, North America, and Australia, birth defects are <52/1000 live births [148]. In the Arabian Gulf countries, congenital malformations are the second leading cause of infant death (2.1–19.2 deaths/1,000 people) compared with the world average (8.3 deaths/1,000 people) [189,191]. Major birth malformations of 7.9/1000, 12.5/1000, and 24.6/1000 were registered in the UAE, Kuwait, and Oman, respectively [20,194,197]. Al-Talabani *et al.* (1998), surveyed 24,233 births in UAE for the presence of major congenital malformations. Of the total births, 401 babies (16.6/1000) had a major malformation, live births (15.6/1000), and stillbirths (135/1000). The perinatal mortality was 406/1000. Classification of 401 malformed infants by mode of inheritance showed the following: chromosomal anomalies (19%), single-gene disorder (24%), multifactorial disorders (26%), sporadic conditions (26%) [198].

The factors leading to the high incidence of congenital and genetic disorders in Arab countries are:

• High fertility rate (1.7–6.6 children born/woman) compared to the world average (2.6 children born/woman).

• High rate of consanguinity marriages, particularly the first-cousin. The risk of birth defects in first-cousin marriages is estimated to be 2–2.5 times the general population rate.

• Services for the prevention and control of genetic disorders are restricted by certain cultural, legal, and religious limitations on selective termination of pregnancy of malformed fetus.

• The rate of children with Down's syndrome in some Arab countries exceeds the 1.2–1.7 per 1000 typical for western countries. This may be related to the relatively high proportion of births to older mothers in the region.

● Insufficient public health measures to prevent congenital and genetic diseases coupled with deficiency in health care before and during the pregnancy [20,152].

Pre-implantation genetic diagnosis is desirable in Arab countries, as it does not involve the decision to terminate the pregnancy. A study in the UAE found that most people are in favor of this type of prevention [199]. The decision to terminate an affected fetus is influenced by a variety of factors, including the country's laws and health system, parental level of education, socioeconomic status, religious and cultural beliefs. Many religions do not prohibit the termination of pregnancy for medical reasons, providing termination be performed in the early pregnancy [152,181,186]. In Islam, the fetus is believed to become a living soul after 120 days gestation, and abortion after that point is viewed as impermissible. Several Arab countries including Saudi Arabia, Jordan, UAE, Bahrain, Kuwait, Qatar, Lebanon, Palestine, and others, allow pregnancy termination within the first 120 days after conception. This can be done if there is no doubt that the fetus is affected by severe malformations and is incompatible with life after birth, or there will be severe disability and suffering that is unsuitable for treatment. It is permitted after 120 days when continuing the pregnancy would risk the mother's life. In these countries, the termination of pregnancy with thalassemia is not practiced due to religious restraints. Only Tunisia and Turkey allow women to have an abortion on demand during the first trimester. In Egypt, the highest Islamic council (Al-Azhar) issued a religious edict permitting unmarried women that are victims of rape access to abortion even after 120 days.

In the United Kingdom, for example, antenatal testing for fetal abnormalities is offered to all pregnant women, but most abnormalities are not detected until after 14 weeks of pregnancy. Screening tests for Down's syndrome can be offered at 11-14 weeks of pregnancy, and a detailed ultrasound examination of the fetus at 18-20 weeks. When an abnormality is detected using ultrasonography or biochemical tests, a woman may choose abortion. This can be performed by either surgical or medical methods. Surgery is safer and preferred by women in the second trimester [BMJ 2013;347:f4165]. Religion plays an important role in a patient's bioethical decision to have an abortion as well as in a country's abortion policy. Roman Catholicism takes a strict anti-abortion position, but this strictness only dates to 1930. Jewish tradition allows for abortion for the sake of the mother because there is no soul in the first 40 days, and even in the latter stages of pregnancy. Buddhist belief in reincarnation, makes Buddhists oppose legal abortion.

# CONCLUDING REMARKS

Thalassaemia is one of the most common genetic disorders worldwide and presents significant public health and social challenges in areas where incidence is high. The manifestations of the condition are modulated by several genetic, racial, and environmental factors. Thalassemia is an autosomal recessive inheritance of chronic hemolytic anemia. Among thalassemia types, thalassemia major (TM) is associated with the most severe clinical changes and life-threatening risk. TM leads to serious medical, social, psychological, and economic problems for patients and their families as well as budget and care burden for the public health services. Children with TM have a significantly higher incidence of dental caries and periodontal disease. Only one-fifth have no caries and more than 90% of the patients have gingivitis. The tooth crown size of TM patients is significantly reduced. The maxillary and mandibular dental arches are short and narrow. Patients have skeletal/dental Class II malocclusion. The pallor of oral mucosa and yellowing of the skin are characteristics of underlying chronic anemia.TM children and adolescents suffer from short stature and underweight. Their tooth development is significantly delayed. The orofacial manifestations of TM are numerous and intense. They are due to intense hyperplasia of the bone marrow and expansion of the marrow cavity in response to severe hemolytic anemia, chronic hypoxia, and ineffective erythropoiesis. Regular blood transfusion is the mainstay of care for people with TM by improving anemia and suppresses ineffective erythropoiesis. Manifestations of TM increase with age. Early diagnosis and management allow a more favorable prognosis and minimize complications.

The Arab population has specific genetic diseases. Autosomal recessive genetic diseases are important causes of infant morbidity and mortality, congenital malformations, metabolic disorders, and physical and mental impairments. Hemoglobinopathies, among them thalassemia, are the most common genetic diseases in the Gulf countries. The high consanguinity rate of marriages and large family structure in Arab society are the reasons for the frequent occurrence of autosomal recessive diseases. The best way to control the disease is to prevent the birth of new affected thalassemia cases. Prevention of thalassemia cannot be achieved unless the marriage of thalassemia carriers (especially between relatives) is terminated, public education and awareness of genetic diseases are strengthened, and pre-marital screening, genetic counseling, and prenatal diagnosis are provided. Today, all countries are fighting against the COVID-19 pandemic, and blood-dependent thalassemia patients may face severe blood shortages in their blood banks due to a shortage of donors. Due to increased exposure in crowded hospitals and weak defense systems, these patients are at risk of contracting COVID-19.

# REFERENCES

[1]     Lukens JN. The thalassemia and related disorders: quantitative disorders of hemoglobin synthesis. In: Lee GR, Bithell TC, Foster J, Athens JW, Lukens JN, Eds. Wintrobe's Clinical Hematology. 9th ed. Philadelphia: Lea & Febiger 1993; pp. 1102-33.

[2]     Weatheral JD, Clegg JB. The Thalassemia Syndrome. 4th ed., Oxford: Blackwell Scientific 2001. [http://dx.doi.org/10.1002/9780470696705]

[3]     Galanello R, Origa R. Beta-thalassemia. Orphanet J Rare Dis 2010; 5: 11. [http://dx.doi.org/10.1186/1750-1172-5-11] [PMID: 20492708]

[4]     Viprakasit V, Origa R. Genetic basis, pathophysiology and diagnosis. In: Cappellini MD, Cohen A, Porter J, Taher A, Viprakasit V, Eds. Guidelines for the Management of Transfusion Dependent Thalassaemia (TDT), 3rd ed. Chapter 1. Thalassaemia International Federation (TIF Publication No. 20), Nicosia; Cyprus 2014.

[5]     Olivieri NF. The β-thalassemia. N Engl J Med 1999; 34: 99-109. [http://dx.doi.org/10.1056/NEJM199907083410207] [PMID: 10395633]

[6]     Perrotta S, Cappellini MD, Bertoldo F, *et al.* Osteoporosis in β-thalassaemia major patients: analysis of the genetic background. Br J Haematol 2000; 111(2): 461-6. [http://dx.doi.org/10.1046/j.1365-2141.2000.02382.x] [PMID: 11122085]

[7]     Borgna-Pignatti C, Rugolotto S, De Stefano P, *et al.* Survival and complications in patients with thalassemia major treated with transfusion and deferoxamine. Haematologica 2004; 89(10): 1187-93. [PMID: 15477202]

[8]     Origa R, Galanello R. Pathophysiology of beta thalassaemia. Pediatr Endocrinol Rev 2011; 8 (Suppl. 2): 263-70. [PMID: 21705976]

[9]     Porter J, Viprakasit V, Kattamis A. Iron overload and chelation. In: Cappellini MD, Cohen A, Porter J, Taher A, Viprakasit V, Eds. Guidelines for the Management of Transfusion Dependent Thalassaemia (TDT), 3rd ed. Chapter 3. Thalassaemia International Federation (TIF Publication No. 20), Nicosia; Cyprus, 2014.

[10]    Olivieri NF, Brittenham GM. Iron-chelating therapy and the treatment of thalassemia. Blood 1997; 89(3): 739-61. [http://dx.doi.org/10.1182/blood.V89.3.739] [PMID: 9028304]

[11]    Vichinsky EP. Changing patterns of thalassemia worldwide. Ann N Y Acad Sci 2005; 1054: 18-24. [http://dx.doi.org/10.1196/annals.1345.003] [PMID: 16339647]

[12]    Modell B, Darlison M. Global epidemiology of haemoglobin disorders and derived service indicators. Bull World Health Organ 2008; 86(6): 480-7. [http://dx.doi.org/10.2471/BLT.06.036673] [PMID: 18568278]

[13]    Weatherall DJ. Thalassemia as a global health problem: recent progress toward its control in the developing countries. Ann N Y Acad Sci 2010; 1202(1): 17-23. [http://dx.doi.org/10.1111/j.1749-6632.2010.05546.x] [PMID: 20712767]

[14]    Hamamy HA, Al-Allawi NAS. Epidemiological profile of common haemoglobinopathies in Arab countries. J Community Genet 2013; 4(2): 147-67. [http://dx.doi.org/10.1007/s12687-012-0127-8] [PMID: 23224852]

[15]    Draft policy for prevention and control of hemoglobinopathies – thalassemia, sickle cell disease and

variant hemoglobins in India. New Delhi: Ministry of Health and Family Welfare 2018.

[16]   Al-Suliman A. Prevalence of beta-thalassemia trait in premarital screening in Al-Hassa, Saudi Arabia. Ann Saudi Med 2006; 26(1): 14-6.
       [http://dx.doi.org/10.5144/0256-4947.2006.14] [PMID: 16521869]

[17]   Kim S, Tridane A. Thalassemia in the United Arab Emirates: Why it can be prevented but not eradicated. PLoS One 2017; 12(1): e0170485.
       [http://dx.doi.org/10.1371/journal.pone.0170485] [PMID: 28135306]

[18]   Bittles A. Consanguinity and its relevance to clinical genetics. Clin Genet 2001; 60(2): 89-98.
       [http://dx.doi.org/10.1034/j.1399-0004.2001.600201.x] [PMID: 11553039]

[19]   Hamamy H. Consanguineous marriages : Preconception consultation in primary health care settings. J Community Genet 2012; 3(3): 185-92.
       [http://dx.doi.org/10.1007/s12687-011-0072-y] [PMID: 22109912]

[20]   Al-Gazali L, Hamamy H, Al-Arrayad S. Genetic disorders in the Arab world. BMJ 2006; 333: 831-4.
       [http://dx.doi.org/10.1136/bmj.38982.704931.AE] [PMID: 17053236]

[21]   Tadmouri GO, Nair P, Obeid T, Al Ali MT, Al Khaja N, Hamamy HA. Consanguinity and reproductive health among Arabs. Reprod Health 2009; 6: 17.
       [http://dx.doi.org/10.1186/1742-4755-6-17] [PMID: 19811666]

[22]   el-Hazmi MA, al-Swailem AR, Warsy AS, al-Swailem AM, Sulaimani R, al-Meshari AA. Consanguinity among the Saudi Arabian population. J Med Genet 1995; 32(8): 623-6.
       [http://dx.doi.org/10.1136/jmg.32.8.623] [PMID: 7473654]

[23]   Brancaleoni V, Di Pierro E, Motta I, Cappellini MD. Laboratory diagnosis of thalassemia. Int J Lab Hematol 2016; 38 (Suppl. 1): 32-40.
       [http://dx.doi.org/10.1111/ijlh.12527] [PMID: 27183541]

[24]   Hattab FN, Hazza'a AM, Yassin OM, al-Rimawi HS. Caries risk in patients with thalassaemia major. Int Dent J 2001; 51(1): 35-8.
       [http://dx.doi.org/10.1002/j.1875-595X.2001.tb00815.x] [PMID: 11326447]

[25]   Hattab FN. Periodontal condition and orofacial changes in patients with thalassemia major: a clinical and radiographic overview. J Clin Pediatr Dent 2012; 36(3): 301-7.
       [http://dx.doi.org/10.17796/jcpd.36.3.45763534u3n44k7w] [PMID: 22838236]

[26]   Hattab FN. Mesiodistal crown diameters and tooth size discrepancy of permanent dentition in thalassemic patients. J Clin Exp Dent 2013; 5(5): e239-44.
       [http://dx.doi.org/10.4317/jced.51214] [PMID: 24455089]

[27]   Hattab FN, al-Khateeb S, Sultan I. Mesiodistal crown diameters of permanent teeth in Jordanians. Arch Oral Biol 1996; 41(7): 641-5.
       [http://dx.doi.org/10.1016/S0003-9969(96)00066-0] [PMID: 9015564]

[28]   Hattab FN, Abu Alhaija ESJ, Yassin OM. Tooth crown size of the permanent dentition in subjects with thalassemia major. Dent Anthrop 2000; 14: 7-13.
       [http://dx.doi.org/10.26575/daj.v14i3.189]

[29]   Hattab FN, Yassin OM. Dental arch dimensions in subjects with beta-thalassemia major. J Contemp Dent Pract 2011; 12(6): 429-33.
       [http://dx.doi.org/10.5005/jp-journals-10024-1071] [PMID: 22269232]

[30]   Hattab FN. Patterns of physical growth and dental development in Jordanian children and adolescents with thalassemia major. J Oral Sci 2013; 55(1): 71-7.
       [http://dx.doi.org/10.2334/josnusd.55.71] [PMID: 23485604]

[31]   Demirjian A, Goldstein H, Tanner JM. A new system of dental age assessment. Hum Biol 1973; 45(2): 211-27.

[PMID: 4714564]

[32]    Hattab FN. Dental and Orofacial Changes in Thalassemia Major: An Overview. In: Greene E, Ed. Thalassemia: Causes, Treatment Options and Long-Term Health Outcomes. NY: Nova Science Publishers Inc. 2014.

[33]    Hattab FN. Thalassemia major and related dentomaxillofacial complications: Clinical and radiographic overview with reference to dental care. Int J Exp Dent Sci 2017; 6: 1-10.
[http://dx.doi.org/10.5005/jp-journals-10029-1163]

[34]    Hattab FN, Qudeimat MA, al-Rimawi HS. Dental discoloration: an overview. J Esthet Dent 1999; 11(6): 291-310.
[http://dx.doi.org/10.1111/j.1708-8240.1999.tb00413.x] [PMID: 10825865]

[35]    Abu Alhaija ESJ, Hattab FN, al-Omari MA. Cephalometric measurements and facial deformities in subjects with β-thalassaemia major. Eur J Orthod 2002; 24(1): 9-19.
[http://dx.doi.org/10.1093/ejo/24.1.9] [PMID: 11887383]

[36]    Sayyedi A, Pourdanesh F, Sarkari B, *et al.* Evaluation of oro-maxillofacial changes in major thalassemia. Inside Dent 2008; 4(2).

[37]    Elangovan A, Mungara J, Joseph E, Guptha V. Prevalence of dentofacial abnormalities in children and adolescents with β-thalassaemia major. Indian J Dent Res 2013; 24(4): 406-10.
[http://dx.doi.org/10.4103/0970-9290.118360] [PMID: 24047830]

[38]    Ohri N, Khan M, Gupta N, *et al.* A study on the radiographic features of jaws and teeth in patients with thalassaemia major using orthopantomography. J Indian Acad Oral Med Radiol 2015; 27: 343-8.
[http://dx.doi.org/10.4103/0972-1363.170442]

[39]    Modell B, Khan M, Darlison M, Westwood MA, Ingram D, Pennell DJ. Improved survival of thalassaemia major in the UK and relation to T2* cardiovascular magnetic resonance. J Cardiovasc Magn Reson 2008; 10: 42.
[http://dx.doi.org/10.1186/1532-429X-10-42] [PMID: 18817553]

[40]    Devlin H, Horner K. Mandibular radiomorphometric indices in the diagnosis of reduced skeletal bone mineral density. Osteoporos Int 2002; 13(5): 373-8.
[http://dx.doi.org/10.1007/s001980200042] [PMID: 12086347]

[41]    Dutra V, Yang J, Devlin H, Susin C. Radiomorphometric indices and their relation to gender, age, and dental status. Oral Surg Oral Med Oral Pathol Oral Radiol Endod 2005; 99(4): 479-84.
[http://dx.doi.org/10.1016/j.tripleo.2004.09.013] [PMID: 15772597]

[42]    Logothetis J, Economidou J, Constantoulakis M, Augoustaki O, Loewenson RB, Bilek M. Cephalofacial deformities in thalassemia major (Cooley's anemia). A correlative study among 138 cases. Am J Dis Child 1971; 121(4): 300-6.
[http://dx.doi.org/10.1001/archpedi.1971.02100150074007] [PMID: 5550735]

[43]    Wisetsin S. [Cephalography in Thalassemic patients]. J Dent Assoc Thai 1990; 40(6): 260-8.
[PMID: 2130081]

[44]    Abdulla HI, Hasen OM. Orofacial structural changes in Iraqi patients with β-thalassaemia major. Iraqi Dent J 2014; 36: 76-82.
[http://dx.doi.org/10.26477/idj.v36i2.16]

[45]    Salehi MR, Farhud DD, Tohidast TZ, *et al.* Prevalence of orofacial complications in Iranian patients with β -thalassemia major. Iran J Public Health 2007; 36: 43-6.

[46]    Reynolds J. The roentgenological features of sickle cell disease and relatedhemoglobinopathies. Springfield: Charles C Thomas 1965; pp. 87-93.

[47]    Papamanthos M, Varitimidis S, Dailiana Zh, Kogia E, Malizos K. Computer-assisted evaluation of Mandibular Cortical Width (MCW) index as an indicator of osteoporosis. Hippokratia 2014; 18(3): 251-7.

[PMID: 25694761]

[48]   Parlani S, Nair P, Agrawal S, *et al.* Role of panoramic radiographs in the detection of osteoporosis. Oral Hyg Health 2014; 2: 1.
[http://dx.doi.org/10.4172/2332-0702.1000121]

[49]   Taguchi A, Tsuda M, Ohtsuka M, *et al.* Use of dental panoramic radiographs in identifying younger postmenopausal women with osteoporosis. Osteoporos Int 2006; 17(3): 387-94.
[http://dx.doi.org/10.1007/s00198-005-2029-7] [PMID: 16331360]

[50]   Pallagatti S, Parnami P, Sheikh S, Gupta D. Efficacy of panoramic radiography in the detection of osteoporosis in post-menopausal women when compared to dual energy x-ray absorptiometry. Open Dent J 2017; 11: 350-9.
[http://dx.doi.org/10.2174/1874210601711010350] [PMID: 28839483]

[51]   Kalinowski P, Różyło-Kalinowska I. Mandibular inferior cortex width may serve as a prognostic osteoporosis index in Polish patients. Folia Morphol (Warsz) 2011; 70(4): 272-81.
[PMID: 22117245]

[52]   Hazza'a AM, Al-Jamal G. Radiographic features of the jaws and teeth in thalassaemia major. Dentomaxillofac Radiol 2006; 35(4): 283-8.
[http://dx.doi.org/10.1259/dmfr/38094141] [PMID: 16798927]

[53]   Pedullà E, Scibilia M, Saladdino G, *et al.* Dental and periodontal condition in patients affected by β-thalassemia major and β-thalassemia intermedia: A study among adults in Sicily, Italy. J Dent Health Oral Disord Ther 2015; 3: 81.

[54]   De Mattia D, Pettini PL, Sabato V, Rubini G, Laforgia A, Schettini F. [Oromaxillofacial changes in thalassemia major]. Minerva Pediatr 1996; 48(1-2): 11-20.
[PMID: 9072660]

[55]   World Health Organization. Preventive Methods and Programs for Oral Diseases. Technical report series 713, Geneva 1984.

[56]   Diwan JM, Mohammad ZJ. Study of salivary IgA concentrations, salivary flow rate in patients with β–thalassemia major in Missan governorate. J Bagh College Dent 2015; 27: 55-7.
[http://dx.doi.org/10.12816/0015035]

[57]   Siamopoulou-Mavridou A, Mavridis A, Galanakis E, Vasakos S, Fatourou H, Lapatsanis P. Flow rate and chemistry of parotid saliva related to dental caries and gingivitis in patients with thalassaemia major. Int J Paediatr Dent 1992; 2(2): 93-7.
[http://dx.doi.org/10.1111/j.1365-263X.1992.tb00016.x] [PMID: 1420101]

[58]   Lugliè PF, Campus G, Deiola C, Mela MG, Gallisai D. Oral condition, chemistry of saliva, and salivary levels of Streptococcus mutans in thalassemic patients. Clin Oral Investig 2002; 6(4): 223-6.
[http://dx.doi.org/10.1007/s00784-002-0179-y] [PMID: 12483237]

[59]   Girinath P, Vahanwala SP, Krishnamurthy V, *et al.* Evaluation of oral manifestations in 50 thalassemic patients: A clinical study. J Indian Acad Oral Med Radiol 2010; 22: 126-32.
[http://dx.doi.org/10.5005/jp-journals-10011-1030]

[60]   Kaplan RI, Werther R, Castano FA. Dental and oral findings in Cooley's anemia: a study of fifty cases. Ann N Y Acad Sci 1964; 119: 664-6.
[http://dx.doi.org/10.1111/j.1749-6632.1965.tb54066.x] [PMID: 14219444]

[61]   Ja'afar MN, Al-Aswad FD. Oro-facial manifestations, microbial study and salivary enzyme analysis in patients with β-thalassemia major. J Bagh College Dent 2012; 24: 52-6.

[62]   Calişkan U, Tonguç MO, Ciriş M, *et al.* The investigation of gingival iron accumulation in thalassemia major patients. J Pediatr Hematol Oncol 2011; 33(2): 98-102.
[http://dx.doi.org/10.1097/MPH.0b013e3182025058] [PMID: 21285897]

[63]   Van Dis ML, Langlais RP. The thalassemias: oral manifestations and complications. Oral Surg Oral

Med Oral Pathol 1986; 62(2): 229-33.
[http://dx.doi.org/10.1016/0030-4220(86)90055-1] [PMID: 3462624]

[64]   Kieser JA. Human Adult Odontometrics. Cambridge: Cambridge University Press 1990.
[http://dx.doi.org/10.1017/CBO9780511983610]

[65]   Brook AH, Griffin RC, Townsend G, Levisianos Y, Russell J, Smith RN. Variability and patterning in permanent tooth size of four human ethnic groups. Arch Oral Biol 2009; 54 (Suppl. 1): S79-85.
[http://dx.doi.org/10.1016/j.archoralbio.2008.12.003] [PMID: 19144325]

[66]   Garn SM, Lewis AB, Blizzard RM. Endocrine factors in dental development. J Dent Res 1965; 44: 243-58.
[http://dx.doi.org/10.1177/00220345650440012001] [PMID: 14242328]

[67]   Garn SM, Osborne RH, McCabe KD. The effect of prenatal factors on crown dimensions. Am J Phys Anthropol 1979; 51(4): 665-78.
[http://dx.doi.org/10.1002/ajpa.1330510416] [PMID: 574721]

[68]   Hattab FN, al-Khateeb T, Mansour M. Oral manifestations of severe short-limb dwarfism resembling Grebe chondrodysplasia: report of a case. Oral Surg Oral Med Oral Pathol Oral Radiol Endod 1996; 81(5): 550-5.
[http://dx.doi.org/10.1016/S1079-2104(96)80045-X] [PMID: 8734701]

[69]   Dellavia C, Sforza C, Orlando F, Ottolina P, Pregliasco F, Ferrario VF. Three-dimensional hard tissue palatal size and shape in Down syndrome subjects. Eur J Orthod 2007; 29(4): 417-22.
[http://dx.doi.org/10.1093/ejo/cjm026] [PMID: 17702802]

[70]   Bu X, Khalaf K, Hobson RS. Dental arch dimensions in oligodontia patients. Am J Orthod Dentofacial Orthop 2008; 134(6): 768-72.
[http://dx.doi.org/10.1016/j.ajodo.2007.03.029] [PMID: 19061803]

[71]   Lewis BRK, Stern MR, Willmot DR. Maxillary anterior tooth size and arch dimensions in unilateral cleft lip and palate. Cleft Palate Craniofac J 2008; 45(6): 639-46.
[http://dx.doi.org/10.1597/07-078.1] [PMID: 18956935]

[72]   Licciardello V, Bertuna G, Samperi P. Craniofacial morphology in patients with sickle cell disease: a cephalometric analysis. Eur J Orthod 2007; 29(3): 238-42.
[http://dx.doi.org/10.1093/ejo/cjl062] [PMID: 17556726]

[73]   Gupta DK, Singh SP, Utreja A, Verma S. Prevalence of malocclusion and assessment of treatment needs in β-thalassemia major children. Prog Orthod 2016; 17: 7.
[http://dx.doi.org/10.1186/s40510-016-0120-6] [PMID: 26961902]

[74]   Amini F, Jafari A, Eslamian L, Sharifzadeh S. A cephalometric study on craniofacial morphology of Iranian children with beta-thalassemia major. Orthod Craniofac Res 2007; 10(1): 36-44.
[http://dx.doi.org/10.1111/j.1601-6343.2007.00380.x] [PMID: 17284245]

[75]   Scutellari PN, Orzincolo C, Andraghetti D, Gamberini MR. [Anomalies of the masticatory apparatus in beta-thalassemia. The present status after transfusion and iron-chelating therapy]. Radiol Med (Torino) 1994; 87(4): 389-96.
[PMID: 8190919]

[76]   Lewis AB, Garn SM. The relation between tooth formation and other maturational factors. Angle Orthod 1960; 30: 70-7.

[77]   Demirjian A, Buschang PH, Tanguay R, Patterson DK. Interrelationships among measures of somatic, skeletal, dental, and sexual maturity. Am J Orthod 1985; 88(5): 433-8.
[http://dx.doi.org/10.1016/0002-9416(85)90070-3] [PMID: 3864376]

[78]   Cardoso HFV. Environmental effects on skeletal versus dental development: Using a documented subadult skeletal sample to test a basic assumption in human osteological research. Am J Phys Anthropol 2007; 132(2): 223-33.
[http://dx.doi.org/10.1002/ajpa.20482] [PMID: 17078036]

[79]    Borgna-Pignatti C, De Stefano P, Zonta L, *et al.* Growth and sexual maturation in thalassemia major. J Pediatr 1985; 106(1): 150-5.
[http://dx.doi.org/10.1016/S0022-3476(85)80488-1] [PMID: 3965675]

[80]    Kattamis C, Liakopoulou T, Kattamis A. Growth and development in children with thalassaemia major. Acta Paediatr Scand Suppl 1990; 366: 111-7.
[http://dx.doi.org/10.1111/j.1651-2227.1990.tb11611.x] [PMID: 2206002]

[81]    Kwan EY, Lee AC, Li AM, *et al.* A cross-sectional study of growth, puberty and endocrine function in patients with thalassaemia major in Hong Kong. J Paediatr Child Health 1995; 31(2): 83-7.
[http://dx.doi.org/10.1111/j.1440-1754.1995.tb00752.x] [PMID: 7794630]

[82]    Yesilipek MA, Bircan I, Oygür N, Ertug H, Yegin O, Güven AG. Growth and sexual maturation in children with thalassemia major. Haematologica 1993; 78(1): 30-3.
[PMID: 8491419]

[83]    Saxena A. Growth retardation in thalassemia major patients. Int J Hum Genet 2003; 3: 237-46.
[http://dx.doi.org/10.1080/09723757.2003.11885858]

[84]    Lapatsanis P, Divoli A, Georgaki H, Pantelakis S, Doxiadis S. Bone growth in thalassaemic children. Arch Dis Child 1978; 53(12): 963-5.
[http://dx.doi.org/10.1136/adc.53.12.963] [PMID: 747404]

[85]    Modell B, Khan M, Darlison M. Survival in beta-thalassaemia major in the UK: data from the UK Thalassaemia Register. Lancet 2000; 355(9220): 2051-2.
[http://dx.doi.org/10.1016/S0140-6736(00)02357-6] [PMID: 10885361]

[86]    Borgna-Pignatti C, Cappellini MD, De Stefano P, *et al.* Survival and complications in thalassemia. Ann N Y Acad Sci 2005; 1054: 40-7.
[http://dx.doi.org/10.1196/annals.1345.006] [PMID: 16339650]

[87]    Vento S, Cainelli F, Cesario F. Infections and thalassaemia. Lancet Infect Dis 2006; 6(4): 226-33.
[http://dx.doi.org/10.1016/S1473-3099(06)70437-6] [PMID: 16554247]

[88]    Wang SC, Lin KH, Chern JPS, *et al.* Severe bacterial infection in transfusion-dependent patients with thalassemia major. Clin Infect Dis 2003; 37(7): 984-8.
[http://dx.doi.org/10.1086/378062] [PMID: 13130412]

[89]    Rund D, Rachmilewitz E. β-thalassemia. N Engl J Med 2005; 353(11): 1135-46.
[http://dx.doi.org/10.1056/NEJMra050436] [PMID: 16162884]

[90]    Cario H, Stahnke K, Sander S, Kohne E. Epidemiological situation and treatment of patients with thalassemia major in Germany: results of the German multicenter beta-thalassemia study. Ann Hematol 2000; 79(1): 7-12.
[http://dx.doi.org/10.1007/s002770050002] [PMID: 10663615]

[91]    Belhoul KM, Bakir ML, Kadhim AM, Dewedar HE, Eldin MS, Alkhaja FA. Prevalence of iron overload complications among patients with b-thalassemia major treated at Dubai Thalassemia Centre. Ann Saudi Med 2013; 33(1): 18-21.
[http://dx.doi.org/10.5144/0256-4947.2013.18] [PMID: 23458935]

[92]    Borgna-Pignatti C, Garani MC, Forni GL, *et al.* Hepatocellular carcinoma in thalassemia: an update of the Italian Registry. Br J Haematol 2014; 167(1): 121-6.
[http://dx.doi.org/10.1111/bjh.13009] [PMID: 24992281]

[93]    Cappellini MD, Cohen A, Eleftheriou A, *et al.* Infections in Thalassaemia Major. In Guidelines for the Clinical Management of Thalassaemia. 2nd ed. Chapter 9. "http://www.thalassaemia.org.cy/" Thalassaemia International Federation; Nicosia, Cyprus, 2008.

[94]    Wiener E. Impaired phagocyte antibacterial effector functions in β-thalassemia: a likely factor in the increased susceptibility to bacterial infections. Hematology 2003; 8(1): 35-40.
[http://dx.doi.org/10.1080/1024533031000081414] [PMID: 12623425]

[95]    Davidson RN, Wall RA. Prevention and management of infections in patients without a spleen. Clin Microbiol Infect 2001; 7(12): 657-60.
[http://dx.doi.org/10.1046/j.1198-743x.2001.00355.x] [PMID: 11843905]

[96]    Holdsworth RJ, Irving AD, Cuschieri A. Postsplenectomy sepsis and its mortality rate: actual versus perceived risks. Br J Surg 1991; 78(9): 1031-8.
[http://dx.doi.org/10.1002/bjs.1800780904] [PMID: 1933181]

[97]    Taher A, Tyan PI. The spleen. In: Cappellini MD, Cohen A, Porter J, Taher A, Viprakasit V, eds. Guidelines for the Management of Transfusion Dependent Thalassaemia (TDT) 3rd ed. Thalassaemia International Federation (TIF Publication No. 20). Nicosia, Cyprus; 2014.

[98]    Terezhalmy GT, Hall EH. The asplenic patient: a consideration for antimicrobial prophylaxis. Oral Surg Oral Med Oral Pathol 1984; 57(1): 114-7.
[http://dx.doi.org/10.1016/0030-4220(84)90273-1] [PMID: 6229706]

[99]    Singh H, Pradhan M, Singh RL, *et al.* High frequency of hepatitis B virus infection in patients with beta-thalassemia receiving multiple transfusionsVox Sang 2003.

[100]   Papaioannou AC, Antoniadis S. Cardiac complications in thalassemia syndrome:Clinical and radiological considerations. In: Papavasiliou C, Cambouris T, Fessas P, Eds. Radiology of Thalassemia. Berlin, Heidelberg: Springer 1989.
[http://dx.doi.org/10.1007/978-3-642-72587-6_11]

[101]   Cohen AR, Glimm E, Porter JB. Effect of transfusional iron intake on response to chelation therapy in beta-thalassemia major. Blood 2008; 111(2): 583-7.
[http://dx.doi.org/10.1182/blood-2007-08-109306] [PMID: 17951527]

[102]   Rachmilewitz EA, Giardina PJ. How I treat thalassemia. Blood 2011; 118(13): 3479-88.
[http://dx.doi.org/10.1182/blood-2010-08-300335] [PMID: 21813448]

[103]   Pepe A, Meloni A, Rossi G, *et al.* Cardiac complications and diabetes in thalassaemia major: a large historical multicentre study. Br J Haematol 2013; 163(4): 520-7.
[http://dx.doi.org/10.1111/bjh.12557] [PMID: 24111905]

[104]   Ladis V, Chouliaras G, Berdoukas V, *et al.* Relation of chelation regimes to cardiac mortality and morbidity in patients with thalassaemia major: an observational study from a large Greek Unit. Eur J Haematol 2010; 85(4): 335-44.
[http://dx.doi.org/10.1111/j.1600-0609.2010.01491.x] [PMID: 20561034]

[105]   Li M-J, Peng SS-F, Lu M-Y, *et al.* Diabetes mellitus in patients with thalassemia major. Pediatr Blood Cancer 2014; 61(1): 20-4.
[http://dx.doi.org/10.1002/pbc.24754] [PMID: 24115521]

[106]   Meng Z, Liang L, Zhang L, *et al.* Endocrine complications in patients with thalassaemia major. Int J Pediatr Endocrinol 2013; 2013: 55.
[http://dx.doi.org/10.1186/1687-9856-2013-S1-P55]

[107]   Aydinok Y. Infection. In: Guidelines for the Management of Transfusion Dependent Thalassaemia (TDT), 3rd ed. Cappellini MD, Cohen A, Porter J, Taher A, Viprakasit V. Chapter 7. Thalassaemia International Federation (TIF Publication No. 20) Nicosia, Cyprus 2014.

[108]   Velati C, Romanò L, Fomiatti L, Baruffi L, Zanetti AR. SIMTI Research Group. Impact of nucleic acid testing for hepatitis B virus, hepatitis C virus, and human immunodeficiency virus on the safety of blood supply in Italy: a 6-year survey. Transfusion 2008; 48(10): 2205-13.
[http://dx.doi.org/10.1111/j.1537-2995.2008.01813.x] [PMID: 18631163]

[109]   Jafroodi M, Davoudi-Kiakalayeh A, Mohtasham-Amiri Z, Pourfathollah AA, Haghbin A. Trend in prevalence of hepatitis Cvirus infection among β-thalassemia major patients: 10 years of experience in Iran. Int J Prev Med 2015; 6: 89.
[http://dx.doi.org/10.4103/2008-7802.164832] [PMID: 26445636]

[110]  Behzadifar M, Gorji HA, Bragazzi NL. The prevalence of hepatitis C virus infection in thalassemia patients in Iran from 2000 to 2017: a systematic review and meta-analysis. Arch Virol 2018; 163(5): 1131-40.
[http://dx.doi.org/10.1007/s00705-018-3767-0] [PMID: 29411135]

[111]  Vichinsky E, Neumayr L, Trimble S, *et al.* CDC Thalassemia Investigators. Transfusion complications in thalassemia patients: a report from the Centers for Disease Control and Prevention (CME). Transfusion 2014; 54(4): 972-81.
[http://dx.doi.org/10.1111/trf.12348] [PMID: 23889533]

[112]  Origa R, Fiumana E, Gamberini MR, *et al.* Osteoporosis in beta-thalassemia: Clinical and genetic aspects. Ann N Y Acad Sci 2005; 1054: 451-6.
[http://dx.doi.org/10.1196/annals.1345.051] [PMID: 16339696]

[113]  Voskaridou E, Kyrtsonis M-C, Terpos E, *et al.* Bone resorption is increased in young adults with thalassaemia major. Br J Haematol 2001; 112(1): 36-41.
[http://dx.doi.org/10.1046/j.1365-2141.2001.02549.x] [PMID: 11167780]

[114]  Giusti A. Bisphosphonates in the management of thalassemia-associated osteoporosis: a systematic review of randomised controlled trials. J Bone Miner Metab 2014; 32(6): 606-15.
[http://dx.doi.org/10.1007/s00774-014-0584-8] [PMID: 24748165]

[115]  Chen Y-G, Lu C-S, Lin T-Y, Lin CL, Tzeng HE, Tsai CH. Risk of fracture in transfusion-naïve thalassemia population: A nationwide population-based retrospective cohort study. Bone 2018; 106: 121-5.
[http://dx.doi.org/10.1016/j.bone.2017.10.016] [PMID: 29054753]

[116]  Vogiatzi MG, Macklin EA, Fung EB, *et al.* Prevalence of fractures among the Thalassemia syndromes in North America. Bone 2006; 38(4): 571-5.
[http://dx.doi.org/10.1016/j.bone.2005.10.001] [PMID: 16298178]

[117]  Wactawski-Wende J. Periodontal diseases and osteoporosis: association and mechanisms. Ann Periodontol 2001; 6(1): 197-208.
[http://dx.doi.org/10.1902/annals.2001.6.1.197] [PMID: 11887465]

[118]  Olivieri NF, Brittenham GM. Management of the thalassemias. Cold Spring Harb Perspect Med 2013; 3(6): a011767.
[http://dx.doi.org/10.1101/cshperspect.a011767] [PMID: 23732853]

[119]  de Dreuzy E, Bhukhai K, Leboulch P, Payen E. Current and future alternative therapies for beta-thalassemia major. Biomed J 2016; 39(1): 24-38.
[http://dx.doi.org/10.1016/j.bj.2015.10.001] [PMID: 27105596]

[120]  Cappellini MD, Porter JB, Viprakasit V, Taher AT. A paradigm shift on beta-thalassaemia treatment: How will we manage this old disease with new therapies? Blood Rev 2018; 32(4): 300-11.
[http://dx.doi.org/10.1016/j.blre.2018.02.001] [PMID: 29455932]

[121]  Borgna-Pignatti C, Marsella M. Iron chelation in thalassemia major. Clin Ther 2015; 37(12): 2866-77.
[http://dx.doi.org/10.1016/j.clinthera.2015.10.001] [PMID: 26519233]

[122]  Neufeld EJ. Oral chelators deferasirox and deferiprone for transfusional iron overload in thalassemia major: new data, new questions. Blood 2006; 107(9): 3436-41.
[http://dx.doi.org/10.1182/blood-2006-02-002394] [PMID: 16627763]

[123]  Taher A, El-Beshlawy A, Elalfy MS. Efficacy and safety of deferasirox, an oral iron-chelator, in heavily iron-overloaded patients with β-thalassaemia: the ESCALATOR study. 2009; e82:458-65.
[http://dx.doi.org/10.1111/j.1600-0609.2009.01228.x]

[124]  Saliba AN, Harb AR, Taher AT. Iron chelation therapy in transfusion-dependent thalassemia patients: current strategies and future directions. J Blood Med 2015; 6: 197-209.
[PMID: 26124688]

[125] Algren AD. Review of oral iron chelators (deferiprone and deferasirox) for the treatment of iron overload in pediatric patients. WHO 2010; pp. 1-22.

[126] Galanello R, Agus A, Campus S, Danjou F, Giardina PJ, Grady RW. Combined iron chelation therapy. Ann N Y Acad Sci 2010; 1202: 79-86.
[http://dx.doi.org/10.1111/j.1749-6632.2010.05591.x] [PMID: 20712777]

[127] Kattamis A, Kassou C, Berdousi H, Ladis V, Papassotiriou I, Kattamis C. Combined therapy with desferrioxamine and deferiprone in thalassemic patients: effect on urinary iron excretion. Haematologica 2003; 88(12): 1423-5.
[PMID: 14687998]

[128] Fischer R, Longo F, Nielsen P, Engelhardt R, Hider RC, Piga A. Monitoring long-term efficacy of iron chelation therapy by deferiprone and desferrioxamine in patients with beta-thalassaemia major: application of SQUID biomagnetic liver susceptometry. Br J Haematol 2003; 121(6): 938-48.
[http://dx.doi.org/10.1046/j.1365-2141.2003.04297.x] [PMID: 12786807]

[129] Karponi G, Zogas N. Gene therapy for Beta-Thalassemia: Updated perspectives. Appl Clin Genet 2019; 12: 167-80.
[http://dx.doi.org/10.2147/TACG.S178546] [PMID: 31576160]

[130] Fuchs GJ, Tienboon P, Linpisarn S, *et al*. Nutritional factors and thalassaemia major. Arch Dis Child 1996; 74(3): 224-7.
[http://dx.doi.org/10.1136/adc.74.3.224] [PMID: 8787427]

[131] Borgna-Pignatti C. Modern treatment of thalassaemia intermedia. Br J Haematol 2007; 138(3): 291-304.
[http://dx.doi.org/10.1111/j.1365-2141.2007.06654.x] [PMID: 17565568]

[132] Fung EB, Kwiatkowski JL, Huang JN, Gildengorin G, King JC, Vichinsky EP. Zinc supplementation improves bone density in patients with thalassemia: a double-blind, randomized, placebo-controlled trial. Am J Clin Nutr 2013; 98(4): 960-71.
[http://dx.doi.org/10.3945/ajcn.112.049221] [PMID: 23945720]

[133] Wood JC. Cardiac complications in thalassemia major. Hemoglobin 2009; 33 (Suppl. 1): S81-6.
[http://dx.doi.org/10.3109/03630260903347526] [PMID: 20001637]

[134] Staikou C, Stavroulakis E, Karmaniolou I. A narrative review of peri-operative management of patients with thalassaemia. Anaesthesia 2014; 69(5): 494-510.
[http://dx.doi.org/10.1111/anae.12591] [PMID: 24601913]

[135] Abu Alhaija ESJ, Al-Wahadni AM, Al-Omari MA. Uvulo-glosso-pharyngeal dimensions in subjects with β-thalassaemia major. Eur J Orthod 2002; 24(6): 699-703.
[http://dx.doi.org/10.1093/ejo/24.6.699] [PMID: 12512787]

[136] Coskun Benlidayi I, Guzel R. Oral bisphosphonate related osteonecrosis of the jaw: a challenging adverse effect. ISRN Rheumatol 2013; 2013: 215034.
[http://dx.doi.org/10.1155/2013/215034] [PMID: 23762600]

[137] Fedele S, Kumar N, Davies R, Fiske J, Greening S, Porter S. Dental management of patients at risk of osteochemonecrosis of the jaws: a critical review. Oral Dis 2009; 15(8): 527-37.
[http://dx.doi.org/10.1111/j.1601-0825.2009.01581.x] [PMID: 19619192]

[138] Kumar N, Hattab FN, Porter J. Dental Care. In: Cappellini MD, Cohen A, Porter J, Taher A, Viprakasit V, eds. Guidelines for the Management of Transfusion Dependent Thalassaemia (TDT), 3rd ed. Chapter 11. Thalassaemia International Federation (TIF Publication No. 20) Nicosia, Cyprus 2014.

[139] Cao A, Rosatelli MC, Galanello R. Control of beta-thalassaemia by carrier screening, genetic counselling and prenatal diagnosis: the Sardinian experience. Ciba Found Symp 1996; 197: 137-51.
[PMID: 8827372]

[140] Cao A, Kan YW. The prevention of thalassemia. Cold Spring Harb Perspect Med 2013; 3(2): a011775.

[http://dx.doi.org/10.1101/cshperspect.a011775] [PMID: 23378598]

[141] Cousens NE, Gaff CL, Metcalfe SA, Delatycki MB. Carrier screening for beta-thalassaemia: a review of international practice. Eur J Hum Genet 2010; 18(10): 1077-83.
[http://dx.doi.org/10.1038/ejhg.2010.90] [PMID: 20571509]

[142] Angastiniotis M, Petrou M, Loukopoulos D, *et al.* The prevention of thalassemia revisited: Ahistorical and ethical perspective by the Thalassemia International Federation. Hemoglobin (Jan): 1-13.

[143] Qari MH, Wali Y, Albagshi MH, *et al.* Regional consensus opinion for the management of Beta thalassemia major in the Arabian Gulf area. Orphanet J Rare Dis 2013; 8: 143.
[http://dx.doi.org/10.1186/1750-1172-8-143] [PMID: 24044606]

[144] World Health Organization. Proposed international guidelines on ethical issues in medical genetics and genetic services, 1998.

[145] Trent RJA. Diagnosis of the haemoglobinopathies. Clin Biochem Rev 2006; 27(1): 27-38.
[PMID: 16886045]

[146] Mitchell JJ, Capua A, Clow C, Scriver CR. Twenty-year outcome analysis of genetic screening programs for Tay-Sachs and beta-thalassemia disease carriers in high schools. Am J Hum Genet 1996; 59(4): 793-8.
[PMID: 8808593]

[147] Scriver CR. Community genetics and dignity in diversity in the Quebec Network of Genetic Medicine. Community Genet 2006; 9(3): 142-52.
[PMID: 16741343]

[148] Christianson A, Modell B. Medical genetics in developing countries. Annu Rev Genomics Hum Genet 2004; 5: 219-65.
[http://dx.doi.org/10.1146/annurev.genom.5.061903.175935] [PMID: 15485349]

[149] Samavat A, Modell B. Iranian national thalassaemia screening programme. BMJ 2004; 329(7475): 1134-7.
[http://dx.doi.org/10.1136/bmj.329.7475.1134] [PMID: 15539666]

[150] Shapiro GK. Abortion law in Muslim-majority countries: an overview of the Islamic discourse with policy implications. Health Policy Plan 2014; 29(4): 483-94.
[http://dx.doi.org/10.1093/heapol/czt040] [PMID: 23749735]

[151] Modell B, Darr A. Science and society: genetic counselling and customary consanguineous marriage. Nat Rev Genet 2002; 3(3): 225-9.
[http://dx.doi.org/10.1038/nrg754] [PMID: 11972160]

[152] Alwan A, Modell B. Community control of genetic and congenital disorders. Alexandria: Eastern Mediterranean Regional Office, World Health Organization (EMRO Technical Publication 24), 1997.

[153] Weidlich D, Kefalas P, Guest JF. Healthcare costs and outcomes of managing β-thalassemia major over 50 years in the United Kingdom. Transfusion 2016; 56(5): 1038-45.
[http://dx.doi.org/10.1111/trf.13513] [PMID: 27041389]

[154] Karnon J, Zeuner D, Brown J, Ades AE, Wonke B, Modell B. Lifetime treatment costs of β-thalassaemia major. Clin Lab Haematol 1999; 21(6): 377-85.
[http://dx.doi.org/10.1046/j.1365-2257.1999.00262.x] [PMID: 10671989]

[155] Paramore C, Vlahiotis A, Moynihan M, *et al.* Treatment patterns and costs of transfusion and chelation in commercially-insured and medicaid patients with transfusion-dependent β-thalassemia. Blood 2017; 130: 5635.

[156] Bentley A, Gillard S, Spino M, Connelly J, Tricta F. Cost-utility analysis of deferiprone for the treatment of β-thalassaemia patients with chronic iron overload: a UK perspective. Pharmacoeconomics 2013; 31(9): 807-22.
[http://dx.doi.org/10.1007/s40273-013-0076-z] [PMID: 23868464]

[157] Delea TEK, El Ouagari K, Sofrygin O. Cost of current iron chelation infusion therapy and cost-effectiveness of once-daily oral deferasirox in transfusion-dependent thalassemia patients in Canada. Blood 2006; 108: 3349.
[http://dx.doi.org/10.1182/blood.V108.11.3349.3349]

[158] Kantharaj A, Chandrashekar S. Coping with the burden of thalassemia: Aiming for thalassemia free world. Glob J Transfus Med 2018; 3: 1-5.
[http://dx.doi.org/10.4103/GJTM.GJTM_19_18]

[159] Sattari M, Sheykhi D, Nikanfar A, *et al.* The financial and social impact of thalassemia and its treatment in Iran. Pharm Sci 2012; 18(3): 171-6.

[160] Koren A, Profeta L, Zalman L, *et al.* Prevention of β thalassemia in Northern Israel - a cost-benefit analysis. Mediterr J Hematol Infect Dis 2014; 6(1): e2014012.
[http://dx.doi.org/10.4084/mjhid.2014.012] [PMID: 24678389]

[161] Leung KY, Lee CP, Tang MHY, *et al.* Cost-effectiveness of prenatal screening for thalassaemia in Hong Kong. Prenat Diagn 2004; 24(11): 899-907.
[http://dx.doi.org/10.1002/pd.1035] [PMID: 15565640]

[162] Bryan S, Dormandy E, Roberts T, *et al.* Screening for sickle cell and thalassaemia in primary care: a cost-effectiveness study. Br J Gen Pract 2011; 61(591): e620-7.
[http://dx.doi.org/10.3399/bjgp11X601325] [PMID: 22152833]

[163] Al-Allawi NAS, Al-Dousky AA. Frequency of haemoglobinopathies at premarital health screening in Dohuk, Iraq: implications for a regional prevention programme. East Mediterr Health J 2010; 16(4): 381-5.
[http://dx.doi.org/10.26719/2010.16.4.381] [PMID: 20795420]

[164] Hassan MK, Taha JY, Al-Naama LM, Widad NM, Jasim SN. Frequency of haemoglobinopathies and glucose-6-phosphate dehydrogenase deficiency in Basra. East Mediterr Health J 2003; 9(1-2): 45-54.
[PMID: 15562732]

[165] Al-Allawi NAS, Al-Doski AA, Markous RSD, *et al.* Premarital screening for hemoglobinopathies: experience of a single center in Kurdistan, Iraq. Public Health Genomics 2015; 18(2): 97-103.
[http://dx.doi.org/10.1159/000368960] [PMID: 25613574]

[166] Al-Allawi NAS, Jalal SD, Ahmed NH, Faraj AH, Shalli A, Hamamy H. The first five years of a preventive programme for haemoglobinopathies in Northeastern Iraq. J Med Screen 2013; 20(4): 171-6.
[http://dx.doi.org/10.1177/0969141313508105] [PMID: 24144846]

[167] Alhamdan NA, Almazrou YY, Alswaidi FM, Choudhry AJ. Premarital screening for thalassemia and sickle cell disease in Saudi Arabia. Genet Med 2007; 9(6): 372-7.
[http://dx.doi.org/10.1097/GIM.0b013e318065a9e8] [PMID: 17575503]

[168] Memish ZA, Saeedi MY. Six-year outcome of the national premarital screening and genetic counseling program for sickle cell disease and β-thalassemia in Saudi Arabia. Ann Saudi Med 2011; 31(3): 229-35.
[http://dx.doi.org/10.4103/0256-4947.81527] [PMID: 21623050]

[169] Alsaeed ES, Farhat GN, Assiri AM, *et al.* Distribution of hemoglobinopathy disorders in Saudi Arabia based on data from the premarital screening and genetic counseling program, 2011-2015. J Epidemiol Glob Health 2018; 7 (Suppl. 1): S41-7.
[http://dx.doi.org/10.1016/j.jegh.2017.12.001] [PMID: 29801592]

[170] Al-Gazali LI. Attitudes toward genetic counseling in the United Arab Emirates. Community Genet

2005; 8(1): 48-51.
[http://dx.doi.org/10.1159/000083339] [PMID: 15767756]

[171] Salama RAA, Saleh AK. Effectiveness of premarital screening program for thalassemia and sickle cell disorders in Ras Al Khaimah, United Arab Emirates. J Genet Med 2016; 13(1): 26-30.
[http://dx.doi.org/10.5734/JGM.2016.13.1.26]

[172] Baysal E. Hemoglobinopathies in the United Arab Emirates. Hemoglobin 2001; 25(2): 247-53.
[http://dx.doi.org/10.1081/HEM-100104033] [PMID: 11480786]

[173] Al-Riyami A, Ebrahim GJ. Genetic blood disorders survey in the Sultanate of Oman. J Trop Pediatr 2003; 49 (Suppl. 1): i1-i20.
[PMID: 12934793]

[174] Rajab AG, Patton MA, Modell B. Study of hemoglobinopathies in Oman through a national register. Saudi Med J 2000; 21(12): 1168-72.
[PMID: 11360093]

[175] Alkindi S, Al Zadjali S, Al Madhani A, *et al.* Forecasting hemoglobinopathy burden through neonatal screening in Omani neonates. Hemoglobin 2010; 34(2): 135-44.
[http://dx.doi.org/10.3109/03630261003677213] [PMID: 20353348]

[176] Al-Arrayed SS. Beta thalassemia frequency in Bahrain: A ten-year study. Bahrain Med Bull 2010; 32(2): 1-5.

[177] Al-Alawi M, Sarhan N. Prevalence of anemia among nine-month-old infants attending primary care in Bahrain. J Bahrain Med Soc 2014; 25(1)
[http://dx.doi.org/10.26715/jbms.p25_7]

[178] al-Fuzae L, Aboolbacker KC, al-Saleh Q. beta-Thalassaemia major in Kuwait. J Trop Pediatr 1998; 44(5): 311-2.
[http://dx.doi.org/10.1093/tropej/44.5.311] [PMID: 9819498]

[179] Marouf R, D'souza TM, Adekile AD. Hemoglobin electrophoresis and hemoglobinopathies in Kuwait. Med Princ Pract 2002; 11(1): 38-41.
[http://dx.doi.org/10.1159/000048659] [PMID: 12116694]

[180] Adekile A, Sukumaran J, Thomas D, D'Souza T, Haider M. Alpha thalassemia genotypes in Kuwait. BMC Med Genet 2020; 21(1): 170.
[http://dx.doi.org/10.1186/s12881-020-01105-y] [PMID: 32831051]

[181] Hamamy H, Al-Hait S, Alwan A, Ajlouni K. Jordan: communities and community genetics. Community Genet 2007; 10(1): 52-60.
[http://dx.doi.org/10.1159/000096282] [PMID: 17167252]

[182] Sunna EI, Gharaibeh NS, Knapp DD, Bashir NA. Prevalence of hemoglobin S and β-thalassemia in northern Jordan. J Obstet Gynaecol Res 1996; 22(1): 17-20.
[http://dx.doi.org/10.1111/j.1447-0756.1996.tb00929.x] [PMID: 8624886]

[183] Al-Nood H. Thalassemia trait in outpatient clinics of Sana'a City, Yemen. Hemoglobin 2009; 33(3): 242-6.
[http://dx.doi.org/10.1080/03630260903039594] [PMID: 19657839]

[184] Rezaee AR, Banoei MM, Khalili E, Houshmand M. Beta-Thalassemia in Iran: new insight into the role of genetic admixture and migration. Sci World J 2012; 2012: 635183.
[http://dx.doi.org/10.1100/2012/635183] [PMID: 23319887]

[185] Ahmadnezhad E, Sepehrvand N, Jahani FF, *et al.* Evaluation and cost analysis of national health policy of thalassaemia screening in west-azerbaijan province of iran. Int J Prev Med 2012; 3(10): 687-92.
[PMID: 23112894]

[186] Pourfathollah AA, Dehshal MH. Thalassaemia in Iran: Thalassaemia prevention and blood adequacy

for thalassaemia treatment. ISBT Sci Ser 2018; 14.
[http://dx.doi.org/10.1111/voxs.12477]

[187] Rajaeefard A, Hajipour M, Tabatabaee HR, *et al.* Analysis of survival data in thalassemia patients in Shiraz, Iran. Epidemiol Health 2015; 37: e2015031.
[http://dx.doi.org/10.4178/epih/e2015031] [PMID: 26212506]

[188] Zamani R, Khazaei S, Rezaeian S. Survival analysis and its associated factors of Beta thalassemia major in hamadan province. Iran J Med Sci 2015; 40(3): 233-9.
[PMID: 25999623]

[189] Alwan A, Modell B. Recommendations for introducing genetics services in developing countries. Nat Rev Genet 2003; 4(1): 61-8.
[http://dx.doi.org/10.1038/nrg978] [PMID: 12509754]

[190] Bittles AH, Hamamy HA. Endogamy and consanguineous marriage in Arabpopulations. In: Teebi AS, Ed. Genetic Disorders among Arab Populations. 2nd ed., Berlin, Heidelberg: Springer-Verlag 2010.
[http://dx.doi.org/10.1007/978-3-642-05080-0_4]

[191] Teebi AS. Genetic Disorders among Arab Populations. 2nd ed., Heidelberg: Springer-Verlag Berlin 2010.
[http://dx.doi.org/10.1007/978-3-642-05080-0]

[192] Tadmouri GO. Genetic disorders in Arabs: A 2008 update. In: Tadmouri GO, Al Ali TM, Al Khaja N, eds. Chapter 1. Genetic Disorders in the Arab World: Oman. Centre for Arab Genomic Studies. Dubai: United Arab Emirates 2009.

[193] World Health Organization (WHO). Medical genetic services in developing countries 2006. https://www.who.int/genomics/publications/ GTS-MedicalGeneticServices-oct06.pdf

[194] Teebi A, Farag T. Genetic disorders among Arab populations. New York: Oxford University Press 1997.

[195] Zahed L. The spectrum of β-thalassemia mutations in the Arab populations. J Biomed Biotechnol 2001; 1(3): 129-32.
[http://dx.doi.org/10.1155/S1110724301000298] [PMID: 12488606]

[196] al-Gazali LI, Bener A, Abdulrazzaq YM, Micallef R, al-Khayat AI, Gaber T. Consanguineous marriages in the United Arab Emirates. J Biosoc Sci 1997; 29(4): 491-7.
[http://dx.doi.org/10.1017/S0021932097004914] [PMID: 9881148]

[197] Hamamy H, Alwan A. Hereditary disorders in the Eastern Mediterranean Region. Bull World Health Organ 1994; 72(1): 145-54.
[PMID: 8131251]

[198] al Talabani J, Shubbar AI, Mustafa KE. Major congenital malformations in United Arab Emirates (UAE): need for genetic counselling. Ann Hum Genet 1998; 62(Pt 5): 411-8.
[http://dx.doi.org/10.1046/j.1469-1809.1998.6250411.x] [PMID: 10088038]

[199] Al-Gazali LI, Alwash R, Abdulrazzaq YM. United Arab Emirates: communities and community genetics. Community Genet 2005; 8(3): 186-96.
[PMID: 16113536]

# SUBJECT INDEX

**Faiez N. Hattab**
**All rights reserved-© 2021 Bentham Science Publishers**